OBSESSED

ALSO BY MIKA BRZEZINSKI

*Knowing Your Value: Women, Money,
and Getting What You're Worth*

All Things at Once

OBSESSED

America's Food Addiction—and My Own

Mika Brzezinski

with Diane Smith

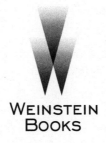

WEINSTEIN
BOOKS

Editorial production by *Marra*thon Production Services, www.marrathon.net
Design by Ellen E Rosenblatt/SD Designs, LLC.
Printed in the United States of America.

Cataloging-in-Publication data for this book is available from
the Library of Congress.
ISBN: 978-1-60286-176-3 (print)
ISBN: 978-1-60286-177-0 (e-book)
Published by Weinstein Books
A member of the Perseus Books Group
www.weinsteinbooks.com

Weinstein Books are available at special discounts for bulk purchases in the U.S. by corporations, institutions and other organizations. For more information, please contact the Special Markets Department at the Perseus Books Group, 2300 Chestnut Street, Suite 200, Philadelphia, PA 19103, call (800) 810-4145, ext. 5000, or e-mail special.markets@perseusbooks.com.

First edition

10 9 8 7 6 5 4 3 2 1

To my daughters Emilie and Carlie

This book is about making good decisions
by yourself and for yourself

CONTENTS

ACKNOWLEDGMENTS

Writing this book has been both wrenching and rewarding as I faced deep truths about both food and friendship . . . so first of all I would like to thank Diane for being a real friend and letting me say what I had to say, and taking it and running with it.

Thanks to all our other friends who took part in what we hope will be an ongoing conversation about this very real public health crisis.

Thank you to Harvey Weinstein, David Steinberger, Amanda Murray, and Georgina Levitt, the wonderful people at Weinstein Books who jumped at the concept for this book.

Special thanks to our wider circle of friends who supported us every step of the way, especially Joe Scarborough, my co-host on *Morning Joe* and wingman on the issue of obesity. Joe takes constant beatings from me on the air, but he truly stands by me in the fight to make our food environment healthy.

I want to thank my boss Phil Griffin for always encouraging me to be transparent and real, despite the consequences. My thanks to Alex Korson, our executive producer on *Morning Joe,* for helping us get everything done.

To all the extraordinary women and men we interviewed, a heartfelt thanks for sharing your insights with us. Thank you for inspiring us.

Karyn Feiden, thanks for your deft touch and vision. Paula Brisco, thanks for your clearheaded thinking and practical wisdom. To Dan Tully and Emily Cassidy, thanks for focusing on the details. Lauren Skowronski, you are always right with me.

Diane and I want to thank our husbands. Tom Woodruff supported Diane's health challenge and pitched in with research, shedding light on subjects from science to public health policy. Thank you to my husband, Jim Hoffer, who worried about me taking on one more project, but who embraced this one when he saw that it would help make Diane and me healthier and happier people. Jim and Tom encouraged us to tell the truth and try to make a difference.

To my daughters, Emilie and Carlie, when the going got rough and putting these words on paper felt a little too raw and too personal for me, you were my constant inspiration to try to get better.

OBSESSED

INTRODUCTION

As I have moved through the process of writing this book—drafts, edits, revisions, etc.—I've sought the unvarnished opinions of friends, colleagues, and family members to answer a question that has troubled me from the beginning: How does a person who is not overweight write about her lifelong obsession with overeating without sounding like a narcissistic, woe-is-me skinny girl with an overinflated image of herself, particularly to those who share her obsession with food but happen to be overweight, or even obese?

I can report back to you that the answer to my question was almost unanimous: you can't. No matter what you say or how you say it, you're going to sound like a privileged skinny bitch with food issues. Oh yeah, and a TV show. And a woman who was born into a wonderful, prominent family and has a blessed life.

None of that suggests any kinship with the legion of suffering women whose debilitating relationship with food actually shows when they stand in front of the mirror in their closet. Yours doesn't, so your opinion is not necessarily welcome here.

So here's the deal. I get it. I am acutely aware of the eye-rolling derision with which many may view my role in this book. I stipulate up front that a good degree of my success in life was gained through my appearance. I did not *earn* my genetic makeup, any more than I chose the family I was born into.

I am a lucky woman, and I know it.

On the other hand, I have worked hard, taken risks, and experienced as many failures as I have successes. I've been hired and fired more times than I would like to recall, have struggled for two decades to bring balance to my professional and family life, have been paid less because I am a woman, and have struggled through one eating disorder after another. But each challenge taught me a lesson I would not have learned otherwise.

The experiences I relate in this book would be no different had I weighed 115 pounds or 215, and the fact that I am closer to the former does not negate the fact that, but for fortunate genetics and the will to change my life, I would be closer to the latter. But if that were the case, I would not be working in television, a visual industry that demands a certain look. It may seem harsh, but, as I wrote in my last book, in order to know your value you must have a clear-eyed understanding of what people are buying. To the extent that I may currently have that look, I am grateful.

So the question is how do I make my point—that absent a fundamental change in the way we consume, prepare, and market food to our children and all citizens, we will never be able to attack the myriad eating disorders that affect millions of Americans today—without coming out and addressing my own internal food issues, despite an external appearance to the contrary?

I'll tell you how. It's too important an issue to ignore. I'll just do it.

―*wwr*―

This is the book I have been afraid to write . . . terrified actually. It deals with an issue that is radioactive for me. How I eat, diet, and look has tied me up in knots my entire life, and I know I am not alone. I have been held hostage by food since I was thirteen years old. My body started filling out more than the figures of other girls in my class, and that set off what has become a thirty-year battle with my body image. Food has been my enemy. My determination to be thin has led me to extremes, and I've done damage to my body and my mind in the process.

It has taken me a very long time to find a way back to health and balance, both physically and emotionally. I'm not there yet, but I've come a long way, and it's time that I have the guts to talk about it. My battle is not over, but I think my story, and the stories of my friends and confidantes, many of them public figures who have had the courage to speak out about very private matters, might help you. I'm going to come clean, and you'll see that you and I have a lot more in common than you might think.

This book is all about the need to nurture a conversation and start turning back the tide of the obesity epidemic. It's time we have a real and public dialogue about food and weight, and the threat they pose to the nation's security. We have to. Right now, the Centers for Disease Control and Prevention tells us that two in every three Americans is either overweight or obese. We also have 12.5 million children, ages two to nineteen, who are obese—that's three times as many as we had in the 1980s.[1]

This book is all about the need to nurture a conversation and start turning back the tide of the obesity epidemic.—*Mika*

Between the increases in disordered eating and the rise in obesity, our kids, especially our girls, are in grave danger. As a mother I know that unless we intervene, my own two daughters will face challenges that might be even more frightening than those with which I have struggled. I cherish my girls, Emilie and Carlie, and I have to do everything I can to prevent them from becoming as obsessed with food as I have been. I owe it to them to work out my own issues and to start talking about what's going on in our society, and how we can change.

I have never told my own story, not even to my closest friends, until now. But thanks to friends who have helped with this book, including the late Norah Ephron, Gayle King, Chris Christie, Jennifer Hudson, and countless others, my double life ends now. The truth is out. It's not a pretty one, but I no longer care. Light really is the best disinfectant, and it is way past time to shine it on America's screwed-up attitude toward food and what it is doing to us all.

One thing that has always driven me crazy about my internal body image wars is that friends and family members assume that being thin is my natural state. It most definitely is not. The truth is that I live under a daily tyranny of food cravings, and I fight against them constantly. I resent those around me who seem able to eat whatever they want, and I resent those who look at me, like my friend and co-author Diane Smith once did, and think, *Seriously, Mika, what would you know about being fat?*

The truth is that I live under a daily tyranny of food cravings, and I fight against them constantly.—*Mika*

Believe me, I know a lot. For years, I suffered from an almost uncontrollable urge to eat certain foods. My disordered eating patterns extended from late nights in high school, when I would jam two or three Big Macs down my throat, to all-night eating sessions alone in my dorm room, to an Ambien-addled night when I walked downstairs as if in a trance, in front of my horrified husband, who watched me scarf down an entire jar of Nutella with my bare hands.

I am finally ready to lay out the truth about all that. But it is really important that we put my struggles with the power of food—and Diane's, and possibly yours—into a larger context. This is not just a story about each of us as individuals. It is also the story of a nation that makes eating hard to control.

Of course we are each responsible for our own behavior, and in the end we make our own decisions about what we eat. But we don't do it in a vacuum. With so many Americans either overweight or obese, something larger must be going on. It can't be that all of us just lack moral fiber. Some of the problem has to be the kind of food available to us, and the environment in which we eat it.

It's becoming more and more obvious that our national obesity crisis is not just a "discipline" issue. It is also an inevitable response to all sorts of forces around us, from the images we have about women's bodies in society to the policies that make it harder for kids to get healthy food at school and easier for agricultural subsidies that put cheap food filled with sugar, fat, and salt within easy reach.

In this book I am going to be talking about all of this. Diane and I will be very honest about why we have sometimes eaten so badly, and we ask that you start being honest with your friends and family, too. Only by realizing that we are all in this together can we appreciate the need to think more about the forces that have put us here. And then we can get very specific about what you and I can do to turn things around—for ourselves, our children, and our communities.

I was in my early thirties when I realized that the way I ate was on a collision course with my dream of being a news reporter. I was a wife, a mother, and a journalist, and I just *had* to stay healthy if I was going to juggle all those responsibilities successfully. But staying healthy was hard when I was behaving like a junkie hungering for the next hit of crack. My mind wandered to food all the time. I can't begin to tell you how much time I have wasted with those thoughts. I have literally spent years of my life obsessing over food, chasing after food, gobbling down food—and then punishing myself for eating too much and trying to erase the effects.

I'm not afraid to say I am addicted to certain foods. To me, addiction is the right word: the one that fits the pattern of my behavior and helps to explain some of the poor choices I have made. Not everyone agrees. Some of the scientists, doctors, and therapists who spoke with Diane and me as we were writing this book are still skeptical about the idea that food can be addictive, because obviously it satisfies one of our most fundamental biological needs. We have to eat in order to survive, just as we have to breathe. In fact, I've heard people laugh at that idea and say, "What's next? Are you going to tell me we're addicted to air, too?"

I was behaving like a junkie hungering for the next hit of crack. My mind wandered to food all the time. I can't begin to tell you how much time I have wasted with those thoughts.—*Mika*

But while we do have to eat, we don't have to eat cake and chips and over-the-top entrées loaded with high-calorie ingredients and chemical flavorings. And those are the kinds of foods that trigger an addiction-like response. In these pages, you'll be hearing from people who are doing groundbreaking research on food addiction; research that is helping us understand what compulsive eating has in common with substance dependence.

Hear me out and then think about this during your next meal, or when you head to McDonald's. Although you might go out absolutely determined to order a salad, you will in all likelihood be drawn instead to items on the menu that are "hyperpalatable" or "ultraprocessed." These are foods that have been packed with sugar, fat, and salt; foods we have processed, produced, and ingested in massive amounts over the last thirty or forty years. They are the foods many researchers blame, at least in part, for making our country one of the most obese on earth.

It shouldn't surprise you to learn that these are also the foods I've been addicted to for years. The ugly truth is that millions of Americans like me have become "hooked" on foods that stimulate the body's internal pleasure system. They give us the feeling of reward that calls us back for more. It's a biological response built into the pathways of our bodies.

There's a reason you don't see people stuffing themselves with fruits, vegetables, lean meats, and nuts. Have I ever sat down and eaten a supersize bowl of broccoli? No way! But like millions of Americans, I have polished off a big bag of potato chips or a pint of ice cream at one sitting. I know I'm not alone when I admit that I have dived headfirst into burgers, fries, and other hyperprocessed foods.

I'm not obese or even overweight, and I am less obsessed with food than I once was, but I still struggle. I fantasize far too often about what I'm going to eat next, even as I maintain (most of the time) a diet that some people think is way too rigid. I know these kinds of struggles are taking place in families across the country, and I know a lot of people are losing them.

How sad for the next generation. Statistics show not only that more children are becoming obese, but that more children are also being treated for "disordered eating." So we've not only got a lot of overweight kids, we've got a lot of kids at a healthy weight with unhealthy food habits. Every parent wants to raise healthy and happy kids, but instead we seem to be setting them up for a lifelong losing battle with food.

—*mm*—

Whose fault is it that America is getting fatter by the year? Is it all about personal responsibility, as the food industry maintains? Or has processed food been deliberately engineered to make us crave it? Could food industry lobbyists in the circles of power in Washington be partly to blame for the obesity crisis that is costing taxpayers hundreds of billions of dollars every year?

Experts tell me that a lot of other factors are also helping us become fat. We offer gym at far too few schools and allow soda and candy to be sold in the vending machines of far too many. We build communities without sidewalks or safe recreation. We have a culture in which every business meeting and every social gathering is considered an occasion for eating. With fast food outlets at every corner, we can satisfy our cravings at the drop of a hat, with budget-priced junk food that is within easy reach 24/7.

Let's face it: the odds are stacked against us.

No wonder we have a crisis of many dimensions. It's a health crisis. In her book *A World Without Cancer,* Margaret Cuomo tells us that 30 percent of cancers are associated with obesity, diet, and lack of exercise. It's an economic crisis, because it can be harder for overweight people to find good jobs. It's a personal crisis for all of us who don't feel good about the way we look or how we eat, and are embarrassed to admit it. It's even a national security crisis, burdening the military

with overweight recruits and a shrinking pool of potential can-
didates; according to our military leaders, one out of four young
people in America today is "too fat to fight."[2]

—⁓⁓—

Remember the days when people whispered about cancer and
called it "the big C," as if naming it bestowed power? Now
we're doing the same thing with weight problems. We need to
stop the whispering, start talking louder, and use the F-word:
fat. We'll have conversations about that in this book, with scientists, researchers, politicians, and friends. You and I may not
always agree about how we got here or where to go next, and
we may not find the final answers. *But we need to take this on.*
We need to talk freely and without judgment about these fierce
and fearsome issues: food, fat, and body image.

**We need to stop the whispering, start talking louder,
and use the F-word: *fat*.—Mika**

I've written on the subject of women, money, and getting
what you're worth in my earlier book *Knowing Your Value*. Like
that one, *Obsessed* recognizes that as women, we need to take
control of our lives. How we eat is a very important part of that,
and to make the right choices we have to confront our body
image head-on. We have to create a personal game plan that
guides us on how to eat and how to live, and we have to understand how that will help us love ourselves first, so that we are
really able to love others.

We also need to be honest about the advantages of being

thin and healthy—an attractive body really does impact our value. Looks matter, and if we pretend they don't, our careers are likely to suffer, which may drive some of us to overeat even more. And good looks can't be faked. If there is a vacant hunger behind your eyes because you aren't eating properly, there is no way to disguise it just by being thin. In this book I will be "put on the couch" by clinical psychologist and eating disorders specialist Dr. Margo Maine, who will help me get to the bottom of my own body image problems.

As I did in *Knowing Your Value*, I will also offer some advice, much of it the result of my own mistakes and the lessons I learned from them. And I'll share insights from my circle of friends on *Morning Joe*, who stretch from Hollywood to Wall Street to Washington, DC. Some of America's most famous actors, politicians, business executives, and writers have generously shared their thoughts with me, and I will pass on to you what works for them.

I want to go beyond the debate Joe Scarborough and I have on the *Morning Joe* set and open the floor to a bigger conversation, a dialogue on how America got fat, why the obesity epidemic keeps getting worse, and how we can turn the corner and step firmly onto the path of health. I want to talk about requiring better food labels and limiting portion sizes, restricting the sale of the huge containers of liquid sugar that we call soda pop, and so much more.

I also want to pass on all the good advice I have been given about how to talk to your children about food, especially girls. Getting that right—knowing what to say and what not to say— makes all the difference. You need to have these conversations with your kids early and often—the issue can't be addressed in a single heart-to-heart talk—and you need to have them before it's too late to have an impact.

Just as it is remains a continuing struggle for me to know my value, my friction with food will not end with the last word of this book. But I am putting this all down on paper—the good, the bad, and the very, very ugly—because I think that is part of the process of healing. If you follow the same path, take a hard and honest look at yourself, and consider some of the strategies for success described in these pages, I am confident you will get there, too.

I hope you will also take this book and use it as a sounding board to talk with your family and your friends. Make it a title for your book club, encourage discussions in libraries and community centers, and bring it to a school board meeting to get the conversation started. Let's push this subject out of the closet.

Talking to women (big and small) about how we look at ourselves and how we eat and how we feed those we love is an important early step. But in the summer of 2011, I learned just how hard having a frank conversation on this subject can be. My tough talk with my dear friend Diane turned so ugly so fast that I thought I had lost her friendship forever. (Luckily I not only kept my friend, but I gained a co-author!)

Diane Smith had been like my sister for fifteen years. When I was scared and alone delivering my second baby, she filled the void and held my hand during the pain of childbirth. We had gossiped together and supported each other through the ups and downs of our media careers. We had shared all the things two friends could share, except one. Neither of us had ever broached the subject of how we battled food and how the very different outcomes had affected our career fortunes.

Diane's weight had always felt taboo to me. Raising the issue seemed like a bridge too far. But now I was going to cross that bridge and burn it down. When our conversation started, I was shaking with fear, but I knew there would be no retreat back to the land of denial.

The "Talk" (as my horrified teenage girls still call it) started on a perfect Labor Day weekend on Long Island Sound, off the coast of Connecticut. We were on Diane's small powerboat. As my girls were laughing and teasing their dad and Diane's husband, Tom, I looked across at her and knew that years of denial had to come to an end. I finally told Diane what I had been thinking for a decade. What everyone who knew this bright, beautiful woman had been thinking but never ever would say . . . until now.

"Diane, you have a problem we need to talk about," was the way I began the intervention that I feared would bring our precious friendship to an end. Diane had given me the opening when she started talking about dinner. "It's so hard to know what to cook when you visit, Mika. On *Morning Joe* you're always telling people what to eat and not to eat. You make me so self-conscious about my weight because it's so easy for you. You're turning into the Food Nazi."

I felt a catch in my throat and knew this was the chance I had been waiting for. I jumped in. "Diane, you think it's easy for me to stay thin like this? Because if you do, then you may be one of my closest friends but you know nothing about the hell I go through every day." Her face turned red and Diane glared at me as if I was the most clueless woman on the face of the earth. As our husbands and kids scurried to the other side of the boat, she and I started to go after one another with the intensity of prizefighters.

"Oh please, Mika! You sit there in your Daisy Duke shorts looking incredible, and you tell me how hard your life is? Why don't you try talking to me when you start wearing size XXL stretch pants—then you can complain. Any woman I know would kill to look like you. You really can't look me in the face and say that you struggle."

I started to sweat. I was losing ground with my old friend fast. Diane had always been on my side. Was I really going to risk this friendship to tell her what had been on my mind for years about her weight, her career, and especially her health? If I was, I would be forced to tell the truth about myself, too—about the double life I had been leading for so long. How I had been tortured by my inability to escape what Kathleen Turner calls the "tyranny of thin" and my own obsessions and addictions.

"Seriously, Mika, what would you know about being fat?" she continued. "You won the freaking lottery: great job, perfect body, and an amazing life. You walk into the room and every overweight woman dismisses you as a skinny bitch. Do you have any idea how women who look like me feel about women who look like you?"

That was it. I broke down. With tears in my eyes, I began telling her the ugly truth about myself. "Diane, I fight with food every hour of every day of my life." Diane leaned in close to hear me over the roar of the boat's motor. "I am obsessed with food. I'm tortured by it."

She rolled her eyes. "Give me a break!"

I was amazed Diane had never guessed it. I couldn't believe that she had bought into the acting job Joe Scarborough and I performed on *Morning Joe,* where he played the undisciplined food slob and I filled the role of the hyperdisciplined health nut. Diane had never realized what was going on in my head when I chastised Joe and Willie Geist and Mike Barnicle for gobbling down Krystal Burgers. She never heard the silent voice roaring, *I want that!* She didn't know I was terrified that if I took one bite, I would inhale every burger on the table.

"Food Nazi—are you kidding me?" I asked in disbelief. "Who the hell do you think I'm talking to from the desk of *Morning Joe*? I'm not just talking to you, Diane. I'm talking to myself, Joe, my kids, and everybody else in America who is tempted to shove food into their mouths without thinking about it. Food that is toxic and is going to turn us all into diabetics. Food that is causing everybody to get fatter and fatter."

I tried to let Diane know I was worried about her physical condition. "You can't climb onto your boat without help. Is that how you want to live? Your whole body hurts and your joints are killing you. Why do you think that is? I am just going to say it. It's because you are fat."

As she stared at me, stone-faced, I figured now was not the time to sugarcoat this health intervention. "Diane, I am terrified to tell you this but I love you too much not to. You're not just overweight—you're fat. You're OBESE. Other people don't see the beautiful person I see when I look at you. They see a woman who looks like her life is out of control, who can't even manage her own body."

I couldn't believe I had called her obese, and neither could she. Diane looked like I had punched her in the face. I had dared to use the word that, as fellow newscasters, we had used to talk about "other" people. I had dared to go where no friend or family member had ever gone with Diane. I then told her in no uncertain terms that if she didn't take dramatic steps soon, her bad habits would break her body down and eventually kill her. "You need to change your entire life," I declared.

I also told Diane what she already knew: that her obesity had stopped her ascent to the top of the media world. I was so uncomfortable sharing these difficult truths that I couldn't even look her in the eyes as it all poured out. I knew how much my words were ravaging my sweet friend. But I also knew that change was possible because I had made real, if incomplete, progress in staring down my own demons. I talked more about myself, finally telling her the truth about the glaring insecurity I'd had about my body for years—an insecurity that kept me in front of a mirror, and sometimes locked in my closet, while my tears flowed and flowed.

I told Diane about the pain and the torment I still put myself through to stay thin enough to go on the air. I reminded her of the time I'd been told to lose weight if I wanted a new job. Back then I hadn't lost enough weight for my employer's taste, so I lost a career opportunity. It had been an ugly episode that stayed with me for years.

That humiliating experience was one Diane could relate to all too well. After all, we are both tall blonde women on TV, with tons of experience and good broadcasting skills. In terms of pure TV talent, Diane trumps me in most areas, and yet one thing divides us. Diane is overweight and I am not. And every year since we met she seemed to get a little bit heavier.

Talking about that with Diane for the very first time was raw, dangerous, and difficult. But ultimately it turned out to be the most important conversation she and I would ever have. Our day took a fateful turn when I realized that Diane had not a clue about my secret self—the one filled with food and weight struggles that were so similar to hers. Diane had no idea of the damage I had inflicted on myself and my family as I struggled alone under this tyranny. She had no idea how much she and I had in common. Really, there was only one difference between us: her eating had caught up with her and punished her professionally. Mine had not. Two different outcomes to two stunningly similar tales.

The very real pain Diane heard in my voice softened her resentment toward me, and the tone of our conversation shifted.

Soon we began talking about how I had won success in part because I had caved in to the pressures society places on women and manipulated my looks for the TV camera. We talked about the mixed messages imposed on women about their bodies, and how those messages are inflated to a nauseating level in the world of TV news and pop culture.

That was the start of a very real conversation that continues to this day.

Eventually, I made Diane an offer: she would work at changing her approach to food and exercise and lose seventy-five pounds, and I would help her do it. I decided to put my money where my mouth was, and to pay for her to lose weight. She could do whatever it took—buy a gym membership, hire a personal trainer, seek guidance from a dietitian, even seek out bariatric surgery. Whatever! I would be paying my girlfriend to start taking care of herself and to change her life.

At the same time, I would work at overcoming my own obsession with food, gain 10 pounds, and accept the new me. My goal was a healthy 135-pound woman who ate a reasonable meal when she was hungry, instead of someone who freaked out when the scale tipped 120 pounds, fought against the urge to eat at every turn, and often felt drained by all that effort.

Both of us would have the courage to ask for help. I would talk to professionals who would help me understand what was happening in my head and guide me on how to clear it up. Diane would finally find the support she needed to get rid of the fat. We would both talk to people who had lost weight and kept it off, and to people who felt comfortable in their own bodies, whatever their weight, and find out what insights they had to share. Together, we would reach out to people who understood that this issue goes beyond the individual and that we have to start making some changes together, as members of one society.

We decided to make a project out of it, which is how the idea of this book developed. We researched and wrote it together.

Our conversation on the boat started us on a journey that we hope will make us both better. Diane will weigh less, I'll weigh more, and both of us will be a lot happier. We're both still working on those goals, but we're ready to tell all—to finally "go there" without holding anything back. I hope this will inspire you to examine your own lifestyle, body image, and eating habits, whether you share Diane's food issues or mine. Our friendship is stronger than ever, and we are inspired by the courage we have seen in each other. It is our deepest hope that these pages will inspire you as well.

Our conversation on the boat started us on a journey that we hope will make us both better. Diane will weigh less, I'll weigh more, and both of us will be a lot happier.—*Mika*

CHAPTER ONE

MIKA'S STORY

If you struggle with weight, I know what you're thinking.

Really? You, Mika? What can you possibly know about my problems?

That's what Diane thought, and it's what Senator Claire McCaskill thought, too. The Democrat from Missouri said that right to my face; blurted it out in front of a thousand people on stage at the Annual Congressional Dinner of the Washington Press Foundation. "Mika, you look so beautiful sitting there in your size two dress. We have all noticed . . . your strong and consistent message of better eating and more exercise. *And I would like to say, on behalf of all the middle-aged overweight women in America, JUST . . . SHUT . . . UP!*"

The crowd went wild.

My outspoken stance on obesity and the way I describe my own diet haven't just incited my close friends. They've also made me the target of online attacks and anonymous bloggers. Trust me, I hear all of you. When *New York* magazine published my food journal, it was welcomed with online comments like this:

> [MIKA] IS OBSESSED WITH FOOD AND RUNNING. THAT IS ALL SHE TALKS ABOUT TO ANYONE WHO WILL LISTEN. SHE HAS THIS SAD OBSESSION WITH FOOD. THIS IS WHAT HAPPENS WITH AN EATING DISORDER.

That reader hit a nerve. He was right on when he pointed out my eating disorder, and I'm telling you, it's not just *one* eating disorder, but many. I've dealt with them for years, and I am still working on my issues today.

―――

I don't know what alcoholism feels like, but I can only imagine that the first drink of the day must be something like my first bite of a Big Mac, especially when I have a second Big Mac already sitting in front of me, and a large order of fries right alongside it. Binges like that were my happiest moments in high school. For someone who preaches about healthy eating, that's a pretty tough thing to admit. But I crave junk food, and for years, through my teens and twenties and into my thirties, all I could think about was how to get more of it.

That's not how I was brought up. In my family, my father, mother, and two brothers ate breakfast, lunch, dinner, and the occasional snack. They ate for pleasure and for sustenance. I ate for pleasure, too, but it was really about emotional fulfillment.

I ate to be happy. I loved junk food and I felt it was the one thing that loved me back. (This was mostly teenage angst. My parents, grandmother Emilie Benes, and in their own ways, my brothers, Mark and Ian, could not have loved me more.)

No one in my family craved food except me. Everybody else ate because it was mealtime. My mother, Emilie, who is of Czech origin, would cook Eastern European–style meals, often serving the wild game that my brothers and my dad loved to hunt. There was plenty of tasty food in the house all the time, but my mother seemed to have her own eating under control. She loved delicious things, but she knew when to stop. She tried to teach me the same kind of discipline, but to no avail.

Despite her best efforts, I was consumed from an early age with thoughts about what I could eat next. *When am I going to get to the 7-Eleven?* (which was conveniently located right around the corner from my house). *When will I be able to get a pint of Häagen-Dazs coffee ice cream, or a pizza in a pocket, or a bag of chips?*

My best friend growing up was Laura Eakin Erlacher. We met in elementary school in McLean, Virginia. "I always looked forward to having dinner at Mika's house," Laura remembers, "because it was what family dinners are supposed to be about. They always had the freshest food and lots of interesting conversation."

The food may have been fresh, but it was also unfamiliar to her. I wondered what Laura thought when my mother served the duck my father or brothers had shot earlier that day. Or venison. *Really, serving up Bambi for dinner?*

One night, my mom made "hamburgers" and Laura wolfed one down. I asked her, "Want another?" She said yes, and I laughed as she took a bite of it. "So you do like *deer meat* after all," I announced. "That burger was made from venison," Laura recalled later. "It was not the kind of food we ate at my house, where a typical entrée was not venison but meatloaf."

I remember feeling like my parents were different. Everything about us felt different, and at the time, I just wanted to be an American. I wanted to eat American food. My mother didn't cook like other moms. I wonder if that somehow encouraged my feeling that I was missing out on something and promoted my cravings and binging.

I found what I craved at Laura's house, and I loved eating there. Her parents had a cabinet I dubbed the "junk machine." It was filled with the kinds of snack food we never had at home. Potato chips, cookies, all kinds of cereals including peanut butter Cap'n Crunch! My all-time favorite was the cake frosting. They always had two or three canisters of Duncan Hines vanilla and chocolate icing on the shelf. My mom made her own icing, but I thought these people really knew how to eat, enjoying rich and super-sugar-infused, ready-made icing. I ate it right out of the plastic canisters, as if it were yogurt.

Laura's parents were always amused at how much icing I could eat. To this day, when I visit their home they greet me at the door with a quick hello and wait while I rummage through my favorite cabinet. "I grew up in a household where there were no restrictions on what foods we could have in our home," Laura recalls. "My mother would buy snacks that children love, and Mika had this insatiable appetite for them." Yes, I did!

Laura and I ended up going to different high schools, but we got together almost every day after class. On the way home, we would stop at the local 7-Eleven and buy mounds of candy and ice cream to eat while we did our homework. Laura could eat a few bites of each one and be satisfied, but I didn't stop until I had devoured the last bite, even scraping clean the family-size container of ice cream.

I don't know why a serving or two wasn't enough, but I always had to get to the bottom of the carton. It would kill me to put an unfinished pint of Häagen-Dazs back into the freezer. Back then I had no idea why I had that kind of insatiable urge. I only knew that if my eating was interrupted, I would fixate on going back for more.

I knew what I was doing was wrong, but it didn't change my behavior. My mother noticed that I would sometimes steal away to eat junk food, and she would chastise me for it. "Mika, you've got to have more discipline," she would say. "Mika, you are just compulsive!" I don't think she knew how true that word was. I was a compulsive eater, and I was developing a dangerous pattern that would chart the course for a very dysfunctional relationship with food.

Here's how it played out for me as a teenager. I was a poor student who had trouble focusing. Junk food and candy seemed to be about the only things I could keep my attention on. I always felt hungry, but it was a nagging, irrational hunger. It was the kind that can never really be satisfied, and it got in the way of my fulfilling my potential as a student and a person. I just didn't have enough focus left to be able to listen in school or retain information.

I know now that I had some sort of a sensory disability, because I retain auditory information, but not what I read. My mother took me to visual therapy for several years, where I was supposed to train my eyes to focus, and I wore thick glasses. I am absolutely certain my academic challenges played into what became an almost debilitating battle with food and diet.

While I have a successful career today, I really believe I could have done much more. More importantly, I could have enjoyed the journey, the joys and blessings in life, if only I had been able to turn off the messages urging me to eat. It was a self-destructive cycle. My teenage mind thought, *Okay, I can't be the smartest girl in school, but I can get that food in me and that'll feel good.* That feeling kept me isolated, even in my own home.

I come from a family of overachievers. My dad was the national security advisor to President Jimmy Carter and an architect of the Camp David accords; he is a gifted foreign policy expert/strategist/Harvard graduate/everything. My brother Mark is US ambassador to Sweden, brother Ian was a key player in the Pentagon during the Bush years, and my mother is an accomplished artist. In our family, intellect was a valued commodity, and I never felt mine measured up. I never really thought I brought much to the table, so junk food filled the emptiness I felt. I couldn't bring *that* to the table, but I could stash it away and gobble it up later.

I looked up to my older brothers, and when they started running to stay fit, I started running, too. Pretty soon I realized this was more than just fun. I saw that if I could run enough I could eat almost anything I wanted, because I'd burn off the calories and control my weight. I became compulsive about that, too. It was like being on a hamster wheel. Eat more. Run. Eat more. Run. Eat more. Run.

Looking back, I think now that one reason I was attracted to junk food was all of the commercials I saw on TV. I bought into the message that happy families ate at McDonald's. Mine never did, but that didn't diminish the power of the message and the images that accompanied it. I started eating those Big Macs and I *did* feel happy. They offered an immediate reward and pushed me toward an enduring relationship with food that was unhealthy and, ultimately, self-destructive.

My mother kept trying to save me from myself. "You have no discipline, Mika! You need to show some restraint." She meant well, but it wasn't helpful. Her words just made me want to eat more, so I did. I got chunky, and my face became bloated from all the salt and sugar I was ingesting. But I kept on eating.

You have no discipline, Mika! You need to show some restraint.—*Mika's mother*

Neither my mother nor I really understood what was going on back then. Focusing solely on my lack of discipline didn't address the core of the problem. With research beginning to suggest that some people are addicted to certain foods, we are beginning to understand just how difficult it can be to control our impulses. Notice that I didn't say it is *beyond* our control; it's not, but the challenge is far from being entirely of our own making.

When I went off to college my bingeing got worse.

It wasn't just sweets. I couldn't eat a single slice of pizza; I had to eat a large Domino's pizza, sitting alone on my lower

bunk in Georgetown University. The entire thing! Afterward I'd
be horrified with myself, but I'd still feel hungry. If I ordered
Domino's with a bunch of other students, I would be upset
because I knew there wouldn't be enough for me, and that I
would still be hungry after we ate. So I would go back to my
dorm room after dinner with the girls and order another one
for myself. As I packed it away I felt a kind of peace, but with
that comfort came a lingering sense of self-loathing.

I made up for the indulgence over the next three or four
or even five days by eating nothing at all. I mean absolutely NO
FOOD. I would drink some water and go for a run. Not a jog,
a run. Ten miles, if I could stand it. I gulped down over-the-
counter diet pills, which made me nervous and made my skin
break out. For a brief period of time I resorted to bingeing and
vomiting, the classic bulimic pattern. Fortunately, my body
wasn't able to put up with this destructive pattern—it didn't last
long simply because I wasn't very good at it.

Despite my eating disorders, I never got fat, but I certainly
damaged my body and pushed the envelope. It was a miserable
way to live. I did not feel good about myself. And I did not look
good, inside or out.

After two years at Georgetown I transferred to Williams
College. (My mother likes to tell people that I had the lowest
SAT scores of anyone who ever got into that college.) I took my
little problem with me. Even now, it's embarrassing to talk
about. Instead of studying and taking in what the professors
were saying, or what the kids around me were saying, I was
thinking, *Okay, I've got to get out of here and run. I'm going to run
ten miles.* I would run those ten miles and return too exhausted

and hungry to do my homework. It was so stupid. What a waste of a college experience.

At Williams I used to gorge on these huge salads from the cafeteria. You may think it's hard to gorge on a salad, but I took humongous portions. I would try and fill my whole body up with salad, along with gallons and gallons of water, just to make my cravings stop. I was desperate to do that.

Maintaining the cycle of overeating, starving, running, and overeating again was exhausting, and it didn't work indefinitely. Eventually, after a period of deprivation I would break down and go back to eating entire pizzas, cramming junk food into my mouth and consuming more calories in a night than I had in the previous week.

Maintaining the cycle of overeating, starving, running, and overeating again was exhausting.—*Mika*

My idea of fun on a Saturday night was to drive twenty miles to the Price Chopper in North Adams, Massachusetts. I would meander through the aisles and fill my cart with popcorn, sweet cereals, muffins, and chocolate cake (I still ate the icing with a spoon). My favorite guilty pleasure was Entenmann's chewy chocolate chip cookies. I could eat an entire box in a single sitting.

After a binge, I would sleep it off like a drunk. A very close college friend of mine struggled with anorexia and bulimia and went to a rehab center. At the time that felt like one step too far to me. I used to think that I didn't need help like the girls who went to rehab, but looking back now I wish I had joined them. I wish I had been yanked out of school and forced into a rehab center. I really was sick, and maybe an intervention would have helped me to break the cycle a lot sooner.

Instead, I just kept up the bad habits. Laura and I were lucky enough to spend the summer after college graduation in France together. My father had given us a choice: study at the Sorbonne or enroll in a smaller program in Versailles. After debating the pros and cons—better French program at Sorbonne versus better running opportunities at Versailles—we ended up in Versailles. It sounds pathetic now, but one of my most enduring memories of that remarkable summer was eating so many of my meals at a McDonald's we found there.

I continued to test the limits of my metabolism. I packed twenty more pounds on my frame, and I had bad skin and bad hair as well. I was overloading my system with calories and nutrients I didn't need. I wasn't healthy, and even worse, I was in denial.

This went on for years, well into my mid-thirties. It haunted me when I launched my career in TV news in Connecticut, where I met my husband, Jim, and started my family. In television, like it or not, looks are a critical component of success. And I was determined to succeed, which made my struggle with body image and the food I ate even more intense. It was part of my inner dialogue every minute of every day.

At WFSB-TV in Hartford I felt as though all the other women on the news team were beauty queens, and in fact some of them were. I met one when I was on the verge of getting my big break. At least I thought I was. I had certainly paid my dues. I'd been working at *Eyewitness News* as a freelance reporter, chasing fires, murders, you name it. I had gone all over the state to get a good story, and I thought it was about to pay off. I was expecting my first contract, a boost in pay, and a seat at the morning anchor desk.

And then, in a heartbeat, everything changed. Instead of handing the prize to me, the station gave the morning news anchor slot to a young woman named Virginia Cha. Virginia was bright and young, an Ivy League grad, but she had no experience as a TV journalist. She was, however, a former Miss Maryland, and I thought that was why she landed the coveted position. I dubbed it the Beauty Queen Syndrome.

Eventually, Virginia and I became friends. She has had a successful career, and I'm very happy for her. But I sure wasn't back then, and that experience only fueled my desperate effort to be thin. I changed my hairstyle, wore red lipstick, and ran every waking hour that I wasn't working. Ironically, in that tormented state of mind food seemed to be my only friend. That set up a terrible tension: when the TV business wouldn't accept me the way I was, I turned to food for comfort, but I also fought desperately against its seductive call.

I eventually got the morning anchor job I wanted at WFSB, and then jumped from the local TV station to the CBS network. But that success didn't cure my food issues. Far from it.

If you look back at me during my first big network job, *CBS News Up to the Minute*, which aired from two to five in the morning, I always look a little out of joint. My face is puffy and

I look stressed. The person inside that body was paying too high a price to fit into the dress size that the outside world demanded of her.

The cravings continued. At times I ate voraciously. Other times I forced myself not to eat at all. Invariably, when I did eat I was drawn to the worst foods possible.

When I worked at CBS, someone would bring in a birthday cake and everyone took a piece. One piece. Not me. I'd eat all the icing off one piece, then all the icing off another. I'd trick myself into thinking it was healthier just to eat the icing because it had less fat than the cake. By the time I had polished the icing off four pieces, I felt physically ill from sugar overload. I didn't understand then how sugar can trigger a reward response in our brains that makes a craving hard to ignore. I didn't acknowledge that I had an eating disorder, and I certainly didn't seek treatment for it. All I knew was that I was haunted by food in a terribly unhealthy way.

I was haunted by food in a terribly unhealthy way.
                                                        —*Mika*

By 1996 I was the anchor of *Up to the Minute*, which required me to drive from my home in Norwalk, Connecticut, to West Fifty-seventh Street in Manhattan. I had to be in New York by nine at night, and then make the same ninety-minute trip home at five in the morning. I was always lonely on those predawn drives home from work. My one consolation was that Diane and I had some of our longest talks at that time, because she was driving from Norwalk to Hartford to host a morning radio talk show. She would keep me awake and on the road.

Only another woman in the broadcasting business could understand what that kind of schedule required. All my other friends were sound asleep because they were people with conventional lives—or at least conventional schedules. At that point I had been working either an overnight or early morning shift for over a decade. The schedule was taking a toll on my body, my mind, and, most importantly, my family.

For the sake of my children and my marriage, I had to make a change. I was desperate to land a new job when my agent arranged a meeting with a woman who was a vice president at NBC. I was hopeful, but less than confident as I walked into the interview. I looked like a wreck. I had poison ivy all over one arm, I was fifteen pounds overweight, and I had developed a substantial double chin. (To a casual observer, I probably looked okay, but in the insanely competitive and sometimes cruel world of cable TV news, I was a shapeless blob at best.)

My low self-esteem and crazy schedule didn't help my appearance. I had a two-year-old and a newborn baby, and I still hadn't lost the baby weight. I had no time to shop, or get my hair cut, or dress for success. I was still running, but I was so tired all the time that it seemed like I was just running in place. And the running wasn't burning off calories the way it used to; it just made me want to eat more.

This NBC vice president took a look at me and gave it to me straight. "You know what, Mika?" she said. "You've got to get your act together. You look terrible. You look *terrible*. You're overweight, your outfit's wrong, and what's that on your arm? Go drink some water, lose some weight, and call me in six months."

I was devastated, because I needed to get off overnights so badly. But I thought, *My God, she's right. This is TV. I've got to look my best, and I don't.* The message I sent the second I walked into her office was "Hi, I don't take care of myself and I am not happy." The second message, if she cared to take another look, was "I don't like how I look." And if she wanted to give me one minute more, you know what that network executive would have seen? That my life was a mess.

When you walk through a door that can change your life, you had better send the message that you have your act together. I did not. So I just sat there, horrified by what she was saying, and equally horrified with myself, because everything she was saying was true.

That network executive may have saved my career. My value was reflected in the visual message I was sending. To pretend I wasn't sending it would have been my biggest professional mistake. To ignore her would have been mistake number two. I needed to learn from her tough talk and take action to become a healthier person, inside and out.

I went back home and took a hard look at the reality of my life—working overnights, raising two small children, and trying to keep a big house together—and felt a surge of self-pity. I thought, *How am I going to do this? Everything is working against me. I'm exhausted. I don't sleep. I don't have enough money for a trainer to help me get in shape or for cosmetic surgery to take care of this double chin. How do I do this?*

And then, suddenly, I had the answer. *You just have to.* It was a pivotal moment in my life. I wasn't immediately sure what I had to do, or how to do it, but I knew I was taking the first step in the right direction. I was *done* abusing myself.

—*mm*—

It was time for some major changes, starting with making a commitment, no matter what else was going on, to set aside ninety minutes a day for me—to get healthy, eat right, and work out.

> **It was time for some major changes, starting with making a commitment, no matter what else was going on, to set aside ninety minutes a day for me—to get healthy, eat right, and work out.—*Mika***

This was a heavy lift because as an overnight anchor in New York City, I was already away from my kids too much. It meant that I had to let others take over some of my parenting duties while I took time to rebuild myself. Call me selfish if you want, but my feeling better and doing well at work was also going to benefit my family.

I suffered the judgments of stay-at-home moms in my neighborhood who shook their heads and tightened their lips at the plight of my poor babies. That didn't matter to me. The equation was simple. This would be a tough time for my household, my children, and my husband, but there would be a better mother and wife at the other end. It was going to take a while—I wasn't sure if it would be six months, a year, or even two—but I was going to change.

It was a tall order for a woman who felt empty at the core,

but I was determined to take control of my life. It began with making significant changes in my eating behavior. I did just what that network executive said. I drank a lot of water—all the time. Water, water, and water. I also started to eat healthy salads, with garbanzo beans and other low-fat protein. I cut out sweet cereals and replaced them with shredded wheat, granola, and Bran Chex. All of that paid off physically, and soon enough I began to look and feel healthier.

The mental and emotional correction took much longer, because true health doesn't come from the mathematics of eating (counting calories, calculating fat grams, measuring minutes of exercise) but from crafting a complete lifestyle that leads to an overall sense of well-being. My compulsion to overeat was still there. I could still eat an entire box of cereal at one sitting if I allowed myself to. Occasionally, I gave in to that temptation (and I still do).

But I was making progress. I cut out foods that I knew were bad for me and slept as much as I could manage. Even though I was still tired a lot, I made sure to enjoy my family, because they put that sparkle back in my eye.

At times, all of this was very hard to do. I sometimes felt as if I was just going through the motions. I should have put more emphasis on being healthy instead of worrying so much about losing weight, but I didn't know the way I do now what "healthy" really means. It was a struggle to meet all those demands that come with scrambling to be a wife and a mother holding down a high-pressure job, and I wasn't looking for the balance I strive for today. I was expected to be Superwoman—at least, I expected it of myself—and now, on top of that, I had taken on the added commitment of trying to reform bad habits and get healthy.

As imperfect as my efforts were, they were huge steps in the right direction. The pounds fell off. I looked less tired, a little more alive, a little happier. I wasn't a beauty queen, but I felt there was that something special about me again, something that I remembered as a little girl, before my body began to change and my eating got out of control.

> **As imperfect as my efforts were, they were huge steps in the right direction. The pounds fell off. I looked less tired, a little more alive, a little happier.**
>
> **—Mika**

Eight months after beginning my self-improvement program, I sent that vice president at NBC a picture of myself looking fit and confident. It was just for fun, my way of saying thanks for giving me the kick in the pants I needed to start changing my life. I was still so busy being a working mom that I had to grab my daughter's crayon to address the envelope. I slapped a Post-it on the photo—no time for a real letter—and scrawled "Is this better?"

Not long afterward, the phone rang. It was the vice president on the line. I had a job on *Home Page*, a new show being created for MSNBC. I was finally off the night shift!

CHAPTER TWO

THE VALUE OF A HEALTHY THIN

MY STORY, WITH JOE SCARBOROUGH, BRIAN STELTER,
VIRGINIA CHA, REBECCA PUHL, DONNY DEUTSCH,
SUSIE ESSMAN, GOVERNOR CHRIS CHRISTIE,
DR. NANCY SNYDERMAN, SAM KASS,
REAR ADMIRAL JAMIE BARNETT (RETIRED)

That experience, and others since then, have taught me that weight and looks affect value. For me, it was literally the difference between "no thanks" and getting a job offer. When I was a little bit overweight and didn't look quite as good, I struggled, and I could see that people with power just didn't have much interest in me. But when I looked svelte and fit and put together, those same people pursued me.

Diane fears that her weight has held her back from fulfilling her full professional potential and being adequately recognized for her value. "As a teen in the 1970s I was influenced by the feminist movement, and I believed that women would be judged on their talents and their smarts, not on how they looked," she admitted to me. "It hasn't turned out that way entirely, though, has it?"

Diane is a blonde, I'm a blonde. She's bright, I'm bright. And we're both skilled journalists. Did her weight tank her dreams of working for a network news program? Is it the reason I succeeded and she lagged behind?

It has been more than fifteen years since I started down the path toward a healthier weight. In the last decade, I have mostly managed to end the binge-and-starve cycle that held me captive for so long. I don't do that anymore. I can't. I have kids, and I have a career, and I have too many things on the line to act so foolishly. I feel good now. I try to take care of myself, and I look like I have my act together. My efforts have paid off in an exhilarating career. Today, when cake is served I usually don't eat it. I have trained myself not to touch it, not to get anywhere near it.

Still, I am far from conquering my problem with food. The attraction remains powerful. I continue to send a lot of contradictory messages to myself. I try to listen to the one that says, *Stay away. This will make me fat. Don't eat this.* But occasionally I am swayed by the one that says, *God, I want to eat all of that.* That voice is still there, too, and I still have relapses.

I have a tightly regulated way of eating because I simply don't trust myself to eat reasonable portions of certain foods. Some nutritionists think my diet needs more repair, and I'll be honest—I am frequently on the edge of hunger. I still exercise to a degree that some people might term compulsive. Achieving a *healthy* thin is a continuing struggle for me, and I expect it always will be. I envy people who are much more comfortable than I am in their attitudes toward food and body image. I wish I could relax my approach toward food a bit. That's Diane's challenge to me, and I'm trying.

But my life is so much better than it once was. My strict approach largely works for me, at least for now. I look at my weight goals this way: I run a business that I know as "Mika, Inc.," and it runs on the fuel of being thin and healthy and energetic. That's the juice that inspires me and keeps me going.

In *Knowing Your Value*, I urge women to send a clear and commanding message about who they are and what they are worth. You can't do that if the message is a lie. For the bulk of my career I thought the only thing that mattered was being thin. I thought that thin equals success. It took me a long time to realize that it's not enough just to look good. That image won't last unless you are healthy on every level, and honest and transparent about what it took to get you to that place. That honesty will give you a sense of peace and clarity, along with the confidence you need to do the job before you, and to be recognized for your accomplishments.

For me, it has been a matter of getting the message I send others in sync with the message I send myself. My outward appearance and my internal sense of self are finally coming together. I feel a lot more sure of my value, not only in terms of dollars and cents, but in terms of my own self-worth. What you see now on *Morning Joe* is a woman who isn't hiding anymore. I know who I am, and I think I look better now than I ever did, because I am more able to be myself.

Virginia Cha, that journalist–beauty queen who took the news anchor job I thought should have been mine, taught me a lesson that has stuck with me to this day: you have to look at what you have to offer and feel good about it, instead of being consumed by what other people do or have. It took me a long time to figure that out.

—

Friends of mine in many walks of life agree that when you walk into a room looking good, you are sending a message about yourself that says "I have my act together." There is research to suggest that carrying extra weight sends an opposite message. Overweight women are generally viewed by their employers as less disciplined, less emotionally stable, and less desirable employees. A study published in the *Cardozo Journal of Law & Gender* showed that 60 percent of overweight women report being discriminated against in the workplace.[1]

The impact on the pocketbook is stark, too. People who are obese have a harder time finding jobs and are less likely to be promoted than their thinner counterparts. And whatever work they find pays less. "Women who are obese earn about six percent less than thinner women for exactly the same work performed. Obese men earn about three percent less than thinner men," concludes Rebecca Puhl, PhD, of the Rudd Center for Food Policy & Obesity at Yale University.

Actually, these numbers might even be more dramatic than Puhl estimates. I have also seen a study that concludes heavier women may face a penalty of as much as 11 percent of their salary.[2] Based on the 2010 average US wage of $669 a week, this would be like paying a tax of $76 a week for being fat, according to health economist John Cawley of Cornell University—and that's provided you get the job in the first place.

Admittedly, weight is less important for men. Joe Scarborough has put thirty pounds on his six-foot-four frame over the past five years and it hasn't hurt his earning potential at all. This doesn't mean that men are immune to the pressures of professional judgment and public scorn, as Brian Stelter, the media reporter for the *New York Times*, understood. Brian began to gain weight at around the age of sixteen, about the same time he got his driver's license. Having a car for the first time gave him not only the freedom to get around, but also the freedom to eat badly. "I trace it back to being able to go through the drive-thru, because until you have a car, your parents can control your eating more effectively," he said ruefully.

By the age of twenty-four, Brian weighed 280 pounds.

"I looked like a slob, and in the back of my head I sensed that my bosses would judge me as a result," Brian says. "I just felt in my gut that I wouldn't succeed as much in my professional or my personal life if I didn't lose the weight. I write about television, sometimes I'm on television, and I didn't like the way I looked on television. And I thought to myself, I'm probably not going to be booked on the shows I want to be booked on if I hold on to this weight."

There was also that woman who turned him down for a date, and unintentionally helped to motivate his weight loss.

Brian started a Twitter feed, posting every time he put something into his mouth. That helped him lose nearly a hundred pounds, and to gain a lot more confidence in himself and his career.

Donny Deutsch is another successful man who knows that his physical condition has enhanced his value and doesn't mind admitting it. Donny is a well-known advertising exec in

New York City and a regular on *Morning Joe*. In his book *Often Wrong, Never in Doubt*, he has a chapter called "The Charles Atlas School of Management."

"I always wanted to feel if shit went down at a meeting I could kick the crap out of the other guy," Donny says. "Now, that's obviously a metaphor, but I think staying in shape and looking good just helps your overall persona. I always say that when you look better, you feel better, and it shows self-discipline."

Donny, like so many of us, admits that his weight goes up and down. "I was forty pounds heavier at one point. I find the times that I am on a physical regimen and eating right and looking the way I want to look, it is tremendously impacting on every area of my life." Adds Donny, "I'm a guy that's been made fun of a lot, because as a CEO I wore a tight-fitting T-shirt." Go ahead and laugh, he says, but he thinks that sends a message about who he is.

"So many successful men are kind of schlumpy. I thought it was quite a feat to be somebody who was successful in business and at the same time focused on my physical well-being, because we all know the time and sacrifice it takes to be fit. I think people look at me and say, 'Wow, this guy's really got it going on! You know, he can really juggle a lot of balls!'"

I asked Donny how he thought my looks and weight affect my value as a newswoman. As an advertising expert who has sold all kinds of products, he knows what gets people to buy something—and those of us in the television business are truly selling ourselves. "Looks matter," he emphasized. "There's a reason you're in that chair versus woman X. The brains and the ability are a given, so I'm not demeaning you by saying this. But in a visual medium or in any medium that has to do with imagery, thinking that looks don't matter and we shouldn't judge—that's just not reality!"

--mm--

Comedian Susie Essman, co-star of HBO's *Curb Your Enthusiasm*, agrees that women on TV are especially likely to be judged based on what they look like. And Susie says it's a no-win proposition: a woman who seems to care too much about her looks "gets described as self-loathing. If she lets her weight go, then she's described as not caring about herself. It's like you can't win."

That's reality, and research backs up this "damned if you do, damned if you don't" aspect of things. A 2012 survey conducted for *Glamour* magazine by Yale's Rebecca Puhl seems to confirm Susie's suspicion. Puhl asked nearly two thousand women, ages eighteen to forty, to envision a female stranger who was either "overweight" or "thin," and then to choose two words to describe her. The most common words used to describe the overweight woman were *slow*, *undisciplined*, *sloppy*, and *lazy*. Thin women didn't fare much better. They were called *bitchy*, *mean*, *controlling*, *vain*, and *self-centered*.[3]

Surprisingly, Puhl found that the weight of the survey respondents didn't affect their answers. Heavy women were just as likely to use words like *sloppy* to describe someone who was overweight. Likewise, slender women were just as likely to say that a thin woman was *mean*.

"What that survey showed is that we judge people who are overweight in very negative ways, and then sometimes we judge people who are thin in negative ways as well. It's a no-win situation," says Puhl, who is an expert in weight stigma. Part of that results from stereotypes of overweight and obese individuals presented in both children's and adult media. "We know that the more people are exposed to media, the worse attitudes they have, and the more prejudice they express toward people who are overweight and obese. That is something that has increased significantly during the past fifty years."

Puhl wants us to confront some of that negativity. "This highlights the need to educate ourselves about how the media and how our culture are shaping these values that promote bias and prejudice and judgment. And we need to find ways to challenge those."

Weight is almost the only place where people are willing to speak bluntly about their prejudices toward an entire group of people. At Yale's Rudd Center, researchers use a tool known as the Fat Phobia Scale to ask people to rate characteristics of those who are fat. Puhl says she would not have been able to get candid answers if she had used a similar scale to study gender or racial bias. "It's no longer socially acceptable or politically correct to say that someone feels negatively, or has prejudice, because of race or gender. With body weight, that's not the case. People are willing to express very readily the stereotypes and negative attitudes that they have toward obese people."

People are willing to express very readily the stereotypes and negative attitudes that they have toward obese people.—*Rebecca Puhl*

That willingness to stereotype reflects a prevailing idea that obesity results from lack of willpower and discipline. It totally ignores the reality of our contemporary food environment, which makes high-fat, high-sugar foods easy to access, and it shows ignorance about how such foods can get a grip on us that is hard to release. It shrugs off the mixed messages we get: one that tells us "being thin is worth just about any price" and one that says "this food is cheap, available 24/7, and designed to stimulate pathways in your brain that keep you coming back for more."

When we lay fault entirely at the feet of people who carry extra weight rather than see them in that larger context, it becomes easy to say unkind things about them. "Blaming individuals for their excess weight is at the root of a lot of stigma that we see," says Puhl.

New Jersey Governor Chris Christie can attest to this. He is often in the spotlight, not only because of his leadership role, but also because of his size. Like any politician, he's had to develop a thick skin, but he's still deeply hurt by some of the hateful comments and tweets he gets. He read me these two: HEY GOVERNOR, WHAT DID YOU HAVE FOR BREAKFAST TODAY, ONE STICK OF BUTTER OR TWO? and THINK GOVERNOR CHRISTIE CAN BE VP? HE'S TOO . . . FAT, AND AMERICANS HATE FAT PEOPLE.

People would never say such vicious things about someone with any other type of health challenge. "It is extraordinary how brutal people will be about my weight," the governor said. He thinks people assume he is lazy or lacking discipline because of his weight, and wonders, "Do they think I got this far in life without discipline?" I've heard Oprah say the same thing, and Diane says it, too.

"For somebody like me who's had so much success in my life, and really been successful at everything I've tried, to not be able to be successful at this is incredibly discouraging," revealed Christie. The attitude he encounters ignores the many complex factors involved in losing and regaining weight. Getting to a "healthy thin" certainly takes personal discipline and determination, but it also requires some changes in the world around us. It is not enough to say "eat less, do more." Or to follow columnist Eugene Robinson's simplistic advice for anyone with a weight problem: take a walk and eat a salad.

"That is the height of ignorance about what this issue is really all about," Christie avows. "I'm well beyond the taking a walk stage. I work out four days a week with a trainer. I'm riding the bike and lifting weights and doing floor exercises for an hour a day. For people who have never had issues with their weight, they can't understand it."

Recognizing that our prejudices are counterproductive is a good place to start changing attitudes. Puhl thinks one reason our biases remain socially acceptable is that we somehow think they might be helpful. "There tends to be this perception that maybe stigma is not such a bad thing, that maybe it will motivate people to lose weight or provide an incentive for people to be healthier." In fact, she says, the opposite is true. "When people are blamed, stigmatized, or teased about their weight, they're much more likely to engage in unhealthy eating behaviors like binge eating; they're more likely to eat more food; and they're more likely to avoid exercise. All of those things actually reinforce obesity."

So we need to get a lot smarter about how we look at people who are obese and how we support them. We also need our families, schools, and communities to protect our children from getting fat in the first place, and to support the work we need to do to reach and maintain a healthy weight. One out of every three Americans is obese (defined as a body mass index, or BMI, of 30 or above) and another one in three is "merely" overweight. With those numbers still rising, 42 percent of us can expect to be obese by 2030. We need to recognize that obesity is not just a problem that affects individuals. Right now, the costs threaten to cripple our nation.

In 2012, four former members of the president's cabinet—two secretaries of agriculture and two secretaries of health and human services—weighed in with a report titled *Lots to Lose: How America's Health and Obesity Crisis Threatens Our Economic Future.* Their report called obesity "the most urgent public health problem in America today" and concluded that "the costs of obesity and chronic disease have become a major drag on the economy." The report blamed escalating health care costs, which are "the main driver of our spiraling national debt," and observed that "obesity-related illness comprises an increasingly large share of our massive health costs."[4]

"The obesity epidemic is jeopardizing our global competitiveness," concludes former US Secretary of Agriculture Ann Veneman, who served under President George W. Bush. I've seen some variation in the estimates of what obesity will cost us as a nation, but a good study in *Health Economics* put the price tag at a gargantuan $190 billion every single year—about 21 percent of all medical spending. If we don't reverse this epidemic, diabetes, one of the more costly conditions linked to obesity, will affect one in three Americans in their lifetime, according to federal government predictions. Heart disease, asthma, and kidney failure are among many other expensive chronic conditions linked to obesity.

The obesity epidemic is jeopardizing our global competitiveness.—*former US Secretary of Agriculture Ann Veneman*

Joint replacement is still another "incredible cost for our country," said Claire McCaskill. The senator had a knee replaced and recognizes that the surgery might have been avoidable had she lost weight a decade earlier. "Any orthopedic surgeon, if they're being honest, will say that a great number of those surgeries are a direct result of obesity. It's the same thing with back problems and the same thing with the big elephant in the room—diabetes."

Scientists at the Mayo Clinic say that the extra medical costs associated with obese patients are even greater than the additional costs associated with smoking.[5] That's a scary thought, considering that smoking adds about 20 percent a year to medical expenditures. Morbid obesity (BMI over 40) is even more expensive, leading to a 50 percent average hike in an individual's medical bills.

People who are obese pay some of the costs out of their own pockets. Under the new federal health care law, employers can charge obese workers 30 to 50 percent more for health insurance if they decline to participate in a qualified wellness program. But in the end, we will all pay more. Working people will face higher taxes to cover Medicare and Medicaid, and they will be charged more for private coverage, as insurance companies raise prices to cover their own costs.

Another harmful impact, according to Duke University researchers, is that obesity is slicing into the productivity of the US workforce, with obese workers taking more sick days than those with a healthy weight.[6] That costs employers as much as $6.4 billion a year. And it's not just health-related absenteeism that adds to their costs; they also have to cope with "presenteeism," where workers report to work, but do not perform well due to health-related limitations.

Ka-ching, ka-ching. The dollar figures keep rising. And we haven't even factored in the human cost of shorter life spans for obese Americans, or the misery of the chronic illnesses associated with excess weight.

—————

The news looks even worse for our children. The American Heart Association says one in three kids is obese or overweight, triple the rate in 1963 when President John F. Kennedy defined physical fitness for youth as one of the goals of his administration.[7] Fifty years and nine presidents after JFK, we are being warned that this generation of Americans may be the first that will not live as long as their parents did.

Dr. Nancy Snyderman has seen the change in her own practice. Nancy is now a cancer surgeon, senior medical editor at NBC News, and author of *Diet Myths That Keep Us Fat*, but she began her career as a pediatrician. When obese children came into her office in the early 1980s, she says, "We sent them to the endocrinologist because we were worried that they had a hormone problem, or that they had a pituitary tumor. We never had parents who were overfeeding. If anything, the reason children came to the pediatrician with weight issues is because they were failing to thrive, and couldn't keep weight on."

Snyderman says childhood obesity has "caught us unaware, and frankly, unprepared for the onslaught of problems." Conditions that were previously rare in children—like high blood pressure, high cholesterol, and type 2 diabetes (which was called adult-onset diabetes until we began seeing so much of it in a younger population)—are becoming common.

And the impact on young people doesn't end there. Partly as a reaction to bullying and teasing, obese children are more prone to low self-esteem and depression, which makes it a lot harder to do well in school. "There have been a number of studies in the past ten years showing that obese students are performing worse on generalized tests at school," says Rebecca Puhl. "In the studies that we have done, kids who report they're getting teased about their weight are much more likely to skip classes and are reporting that their grades are harmed by this."

Bullying can start as early as preschool and continue for years. At first, researchers assumed that obese students were performing worse because they had some sort of learning challenges, but it turned out to be a response to the cruelty of their peers. "If we look at the teasing and bullying relationship, no wonder these kids aren't performing well," Puhl explains. "They have no support, they're facing relentless teasing, and they can't function at school."

In one survey Puhl asked fifteen hundred Connecticut high school students why kids are teased or bullied at school.[8] Out of ten options, body weight ranked number one. "It was ahead of sexual orientation, it was ahead of race, it was ahead of everything else," she reports. "The consequences for these kids are devastating. Kids who are teased about their weight are two to three times more likely to engage in suicidal thoughts and behaviors, compared to their overweight peers who are not teased."

As fat children grow into fat young men and women, we also face a national security challenge unlike any we have seen before. Mission: Readiness, an organization of retired senior military officers committed to supporting smart investments in America's children, calculates that 9 million young people ages seventeen to twenty-seven are "too fat to fight"; that is, too heavy to be accepted into the military. That's more than one-quarter of that age group. According to Sam Kass, the senior policy advisor for healthy food initiatives in the Obama White House, delivering a keynote address at a CDC (Center for Disease Control and Prevention) conference, "Obesity may be our nation's greatest national security threat."[9] It's the number one disqualification for military service.

That's especially troubling because the military has already become more selective in its recruiting than it used to be. "It's not the old paradigm of anybody can be in the military," according to Rear Admiral Jamie Barnett (retired). The military has gone high tech, and it "increasingly needs people who can handle complex systems: sensors, weapons, aircraft, submarines. Now we have to have really smart people, and here's a whole category of people who are smart and who want to serve who can't get in because of the weight barrier."

Ultimately, Barnett says, the nation could face a situation where it simply doesn't have the people it needs, particularly in specialty areas of the military. "We have to address this," he emphasized. Otherwise, the military will lose out on much-needed talent, the nation will lose out on the protection it needs, and whole groups of young people will lose opportunities for well-paying, secure jobs.

"There's significant research that the rise of the middle class after World War II was in large part due to GI benefits: education, housing, things like that. Now we have a huge number of young people who won't even get a shot at that," warns Barnett. "It may take a while to understand what that means for America."

—*mm*—

I'm completely on board with what all of these findings suggest—that there is real value in being thin. But hitting that target is not going to be easy, not for us as a nation, and not for any of us individually. I get angry when I see weight-loss commercials with women holding jeans that are ten sizes too large for them and saying, "This used to be me." They throw the jeans off to the side and show a newly slim body to the camera. Everything is now just perfect. In all our media we are bombarded by messages that seem to say, "This is how easy it is. Follow this diet and you'll be happy." Take it from me: maintaining a healthy weight *is a lot of work, and it is forever. Constant.* It's difficult.

We are not "done" after we lose the pounds. It's not as though we can finish the dieting process and then just start eating again. It doesn't work that way. Obesity experts will tell you that losing weight is difficult; keeping it off is nearly impossible for many people. That's why we need to be much more strategic about how we address this difficulty. And we need to do it together.

It begins with sharing our stories, both the ones that show the value of being thin and the ones that reveal just how hard that is. As a country, a community, and a family, we have to be open about all of this. We should be able to talk about obesity just as we talk about smoking or diabetes or heart disease or cancer. When we see someone who has cancer, we don't think, *Oh, they're undisciplined, they did something wrong.* We feel sympathy, and we want to help.

We need to bring the same compassion to obesity. We can't spend so much time judging people; it's not fair, and it doesn't get us anywhere. And it doesn't help to keep blaming and shaming ourselves either.

Instead, we have to have real conversations, just as I did with my friend Diane.

CHAPTER THREE

DIANE'S STORY

Diane saw my daughter Carlie before I did.

My husband, Jim, was out of town when Carlie decided it was time to be born. Jim and Diane had been colleagues when he was a news anchor and reporter at WTNH-TV in Connecticut. I was in a panic when I called Diane in the middle of the night to say I was in labor and needed help.

Diane met me at the hospital. After sixteen hours of labor, the doctor said, "It's still going to be awhile," and left the hospital to pick up a pizza. Moments later, I told Diane, "I think it's time for me to push." Her answer: "Close your legs and hang on while I get a nurse." It didn't work out that way. Five minutes later, my friend had a view of me only a medical professional should ever have as she caught my baby.

What can tie two women together more than that? We had forged a bond through the pain, emotion, and exhilaration that comes with bringing a beautiful new life into the world. And since then we have been the closest of confidantes. Nothing has been off the table about our marriages, our families, and the ups and downs of our careers. The only topic we ever skirted was weight and food, despite the huge role it played in both of our lives.

When we first met, Diane was probably about a size 12. She wasn't skinny, but she was a tall, blonde beauty. Over the next few years I watched her weight steadily climb, as Diane gradually went from statuesque to obese. Every time she lost a few pounds she seemed to put them right back on, plus a little more. Whenever we got together, I couldn't help but notice the change. It seemed as though Diane was sabotaging her TV career. I remember thinking to myself, *Why is she letting this go on?*

I remember thinking to myself, *Why is she letting this go on?—Mika*

Diane is smart, driven, and competent. I mean, this is one talented woman: she's earned several Emmy awards, has been recognized by the National Academy of Television Arts and Sciences for lifetime achievement, and has been honored by the Connecticut Women's Hall of Fame. A TV news anchor, reporter, radio talk show host, documentary producer, and author of six previous books, she has been on the air in Connecticut for more than twenty-five years. But I doubted other people were seeing all that when they looked at her. Given what I have learned about the value of being thin, I'd guess her weight was making them think instead, *This woman doesn't*

*have it together. She doesn't even have the discipline to lose weight
and get in shape.*

And that's basically what I said on that beautiful afternoon on Long Island Sound when I came clean about how I felt.
At first, it looked like it was going to turn into a very turbulent
day for a treasured friendship. I wasn't sure she would ever
speak to me again.

I told Diane, "I don't really think that you are sitting
around eating all day, but I do think you need to break your
cycle of depending on fattening foods and start believing in
yourself again. You're not really hiding anything with all those
black pantsuits. Everyone knows you have a weight issue."

Telling Diane the truth about her weight, and using that
toxic word *obese* to describe her, was one of the hardest things
I'd ever done. I certainly didn't do it to be a bitch, even if some
people might have thought so. I did it because I want her in my
life, and I was worried about her health. I also thought it was
only fair for Diane to hear it from a friend. It's what other people were thinking when she was on TV or when she got up on
stage to give a speech.

If you are wondering, *Why tell her the truth?*, maybe that
isn't the right question. Considering how long it took me to
raise the topic of weight, and what it was doing to her personally and professionally, it might be more helpful to ask, *Why
didn't you say this ten years ago, when her weight was just becoming a problem? Why did you avoid it?*

I wish now that I had talked to Diane much sooner. It
would have been a lot easier for both of us.

When Diane took me up on the challenge to lose seventy-
five pounds and we decided to write this book together, at first

she was reluctant to tell her own story. But eventually we both decided that baring our souls was the way to set an example for others. No one is better off with silence. As Diane put it, "If we can start a dialogue between the two of us, maybe we can instigate a wider discussion. A national discussion. So I'm all in."

Here is more about how Diane has experienced the struggle against food and overweight, in her own words.

Although Mika and I got to know each other a little while working as news anchors and reporters at rival stations in Connecticut, we really bonded when she was in labor with Carlie. That was one of the most profound experiences of my life. I don't have kids, and my sisters live far away, so it was truly a once-in-a lifetime event; something I have never shared with anyone else.

No wonder Mika has remained special to me all these years later. But I have to be honest. She's a little nuts. When she wanted to know if I would step in for her husband, Jim, if she went into labor while he was out of town, did she call me and ask for my help? Did she drop by the house? No, she ran into my husband, Tom, at a coffee bar one Sunday morning and asked him to run it by me.

She was still a couple of weeks away from her due date when I said yes. What I was really figuring was, What are the chances the baby will come while Jim is out of town? *Yeah, right. I didn't give the possibility of coaching her through labor much thought after that. The only thing I did think about was how Mika looked during her pregnancy, and that was sure frustrating to me. Even at nine months' pregnant, she was thinner than I was. In those days, I was always thinking,* What the hell can I wear that won't make me look so fat?

A few days after I agreed to be her backup labor coach, Mika dropped a couple of books in my mailbox, including What to Expect When You're Expecting. *The books were still in the mailbox when she called our house Friday night. Jim was on a plane to New Orleans, and Tom and I had just polished off a pizza and a bottle of wine. "I think my water broke," she whispered into the phone.*

YOU THINK? WHAT? YOU'VE HAD A BABY BEFORE, NOT ME! WHAT DO YOU MEAN YOU THINK???

I ran out to the mailbox to get the books so I could skim through the chapters on labor and delivery while I stayed on the phone with her.

"Yep, it's starting," she said. "You two should get some sleep and I'll call you later."

SLEEP? ARE YOU KIDDING?

Tom and I lay on our bed, suddenly and completely sober, fully dressed and ready to go. When the phone rang again, we phoned the doctor and headed for the hospital. Mika's mom stayed behind to watch her daughter, little Emilie.

We couldn't reach Jim, so all that night and the next day it was Mika and me in the shadowy labor room. The nurse came in a few times to check on her and told us to get some rest, but like kids at a sleepover, we kept right on talking.

There were a few times I had to step up, like when the anesthesiologist asked Mika whether she wanted an epidural. "Did you have one last time?" I asked her. "No," she said. "But maybe that was a mistake."

"You're on my watch now, and you're having the drugs," I told her and ordered the epidural.

After hours and hours of chatting about everything except how to deliver a baby, Mika decided it was time. I was afraid to tell her the doctor had just gone out for lunch, but luckily the nurse had been delivering babies for years. She told me to "get ready to catch," and three pushes later there was Carlie, absolutely the most beautiful thing I had ever laid eyes on.

As Carlie started to cry, Mika asked me to phone her dad, the astonishingly imposing Zbigniew Brzezinski. I blubbered a bit to him, then handed Mika the phone. In the most composed voice, she said, "Dad, you have another granddaughter."

Mika showed me a lot about her character during the hours she was in labor, and vice versa. She came to see me as a big sister, the "adult" in our relationship. I recognized her strength. In the years to come, no matter what happened in her work or her personal life, she could count on me to have her back.

Now, fourteen years later, Mika and I have had a role reversal. It began with that punch-in-the face moment on my boat. The words still echo in my mind. Mika said, "Diane, you're not just overweight, you're fat. You're obese." I couldn't believe the word she had used to describe me: obese. Who says that to a friend? Who says that to any-one? I was angry and defensive.

My first thoughts were, Oh, Mika, come on. I know I'm huge. My metabolism is shot. I try to diet but nothing works any-more. How could you know what it's like? You and your tiny body in size 2 dresses. Please! You have been picture-perfect ever since I have known you, and when something is just a little off, like your imaginary double chin, you run to a plastic surgeon to fix it. You don't get it. You naturally skinny women think

women like me are a bunch of slobs sitting around eating bonbons all day. That is such garbage.

But then Mika told me something that changed everything.

*"Naturally skinny? No way," she shot back at me. "I do get it,
I get it a lot more than you think. I'm not kidding, Diane—food takes
up way too much of my time and my psychic space. Here's my truth:
I am an addict. I think about food all day long. I am always wondering if I can sneak away and grab some fast food or something
sweet. But I don't. I don't because my career depends on winning my
fight to stay rail-thin. But I know it's unhealthy, and I hate every second of it!"*

*As she launched into the tale of her fight with food, my anger
dissolved. I couldn't believe it, but she began to tell a story that was
just like mine; a story of rarely feeling in control around food. Of
going to parties and eyeing the buffet first, then trying to hurry
through a conversation with her mouth watering. Of wondering what
people would say, or think, if they saw her go back for more.*

**You naturally skinny women think women like me
are a bunch of slobs sitting around eating bonbons
all day. That is such garbage.—Diane**

*It was a story I could barely believe as I looked at her slender
body, but I knew it was true when I looked into her eyes. "I am a junk
food addict," Mika said. She talked about stuffing herself with chips
and ice cream in prep school, gorging on pizza in college, and scarfing
down entire boxes of kids' cereal at a sitting. That habit caused her
husband, Jim, to nickname her "Jethro," after the Beverly Hillbil-
lies character with the enormous appetite. I really could not imagine
her acting that way. I'd never seen it.*

Mika's honesty about herself helped me hear what else she was trying to say.

"You're fat," Mika blurted. "If you don't lose the weight now, you're going to die. Plain and simple: your weight will kill you." That was either the rudest thing anyone had ever said to me, or the kindest. That's Mika. She's no diplomat. She puts all her cards on the table, and she was characteristically blunt. "I love you Diane, and you are fat," she said.

Friends, family, and colleagues had been dancing around my dramatic weight gain over the last ten years, so it was shocking to hear it stated so bluntly. Mika softened it a little when she said, "I want you to be around for my girls. They need another woman in their lives, especially when I am driving them nuts." That last part made me laugh, because it's true!

Up until then I had always thought about my weight as an issue of vanity. When I was heavy I didn't look the way I wanted to look, or how TV viewers expected me to look. I never really considered my weight to be a health issue, although I should have. My dad was a skinny kid and a slender young adult, but he has been overweight since then, and heart disease very nearly killed him. It's a medical miracle and a testament to his constitution that he's still around. My grandmother was overweight and later in life developed diabetes, which she called her "sugar problem." At the time, I didn't recognize the link between diabetes and obesity, but I sure do now.

I was moving along the same path. A path that was almost guaranteed to result in one or more chronic diseases.

—⁓—

Shortly after our infamous encounter on Long Island Sound, I suggested to Mika that she write a book about her struggles with food. Readers have told her how much they have learned from her earlier books, about finding life and work balance, and about learning to stand up for yourself in the workplace, and knowing your true value. I thought if Mika told her own story, it would help other women.

Mika took me up on the idea of writing this book, but I had no idea she was planning to aim her message squarely at me. And then my cell phone rang as I was driving to a speaking engagement in the far west corner of Connecticut, about ninety minutes from where I live. Mika was on the line. It was nearly dusk and I was heading down a lonely country road, not feeling great about giving the speech.

I'm a former radio talk show host and I love talking to people, but for several years the fun of greeting a live audience and spending a couple of hours with them had disappeared. Instead of looking forward to it I'd been feeling a kind of dread, because I knew the audience wouldn't see the person they expected, that stylish, slender anchorwoman of years ago. Instead, they would face a fat, fiftyish female who felt frumpy in a size 18 jacket and stretchy pants. You can hide some of that on TV with good camera work, but standing at the microphone at the front of the room, they were going to see all of me.

On top of that my feet hurt, my knees ached, and I dreaded having to stand at a podium during my talk. It was going to take all the charm I could muster to make them forget who and what they were looking at, and concentrate instead on what I was saying. I wanted to get them wrapped up in my stories: stories about the people and places that make the state of Connecticut special, and give it character and heart. Those are the stories I had reported on TV and radio, and had written books about for years. Sharing them was my passion.

But that sharing was getting harder and harder to do because of my weight. I hated the way I looked in person and on the screen. I won an Emmy for a documentary I produced and hosted a couple of years ago, but I couldn't even watch myself on TV because I couldn't stand how fat I looked.

I couldn't seem to do much about it. I had dieted on and off all my life, and nothing seemed to work. During my TV news career I was a size 10 at my thinnest, and more often a lot bigger than that. I was always the largest woman in the television newsroom, always worried about how I would look on camera when I had to step out from behind the desk. My first reaction when I got invited to a big event was always, What the hell am I going to wear? How much weight can I lose before then so I will fit into something nice? And then the diet cycle would start all over again.

I can barely remember a time when I wasn't worried about how I looked and what people were thinking. I knew I was smarter and more talented than many of my peers, but I just couldn't conquer my weight. No one had ever said it, but I could imagine what people were thinking: Why doesn't she get it together and lose the weight?

———

As soon as I answered Mika's call, she launched into her proposal. She asked me to write a book with her, but the offer came with a catch. I had to set a goal of losing seventy-five pounds as we worked on the book project. She promised to pay for whatever treatments would help, and to be my cheerleader every step of the way, but I had to make the commitment.

As Mika outlined her idea, I started to cry. "Diane," she told me, "this is it: no more excuses. You have got to lose the weight. I know you don't want to hear it, but you must. Let's make a deal. I'll pay you to write this book with me. We will talk about everything, and when we are finished, we will both be better off. You'll be thin and healthy, and I will be in a better place in my mind. But you have to lose A TON of weight . . . Come on, let's do it."

I choked up as she plowed ahead with her characteristic insistence. Mika can be hard to turn down, but it was daunting to consider how tough it would be. My eyes were red and my mascara a little runny when I finally pulled into the place where I was giving my speech, but I had made up my mind. I was going to take Mika up on the offer. I knew it could be my last serious shot at getting my life back, and regaining what fat had taken away from me.

Have you ever watched those weight-loss commercials with celebrities like Valerie Bertinelli and Jennifer Hudson and said to yourself, Yeah I bet I could lose weight if someone paid me to do it. I know I have. Now someone was making me that offer. I really couldn't say no. How would I face my sisters if they found out I had turned Mika down? Especially Suzanne, who had cheered her friend Valerie Bertinelli through her own weight-loss battle. But I had SO much weight to lose, and at my age (the mid-fifties), could I really do it? All I knew was that I had to try. As cutting as Mika's words had been when we first went down this path together, I knew they were driven by love. She was right; it had gotten that bad. I was having trouble getting onto our small boat, trouble getting into the bathtub.

I had given up shopping because nothing ever fit, and plus-size clothes are just not that attractive on me. I now dressed for what fit and covered the most sins, not for what looked good. I was losing my self-confidence. The media business is tough enough for women without the added obstacle of being fat.

I now dressed for what fit and covered the most sins, not for what looked good. I was losing my self-confidence.—Diane

Still, the idea of sharing my feelings about my struggles with weight made me a little sick to my stomach. It was hard enough to talk to Mika about it, much less to everyone who would read the book. Did she have any idea how difficult it was going to be for me? How embarrassing? Is this bargain we're making brilliant or just plain crazy? Is it even possible?

As a TV personality and a radio talk show host, I've always emphasized the bright, the light, and the positive. Every inch of me resists admitting how bad I feel about my weight. But Mika is adamant that we begin the conversation, and she insists that I not hold back. No one knows more than I do how hard that's going to be, but here goes.

—————

Dieting is the most active sport I have ever engaged in. If practice made perfect, I'd be thin as a ghost. Honestly, I have been dieting almost all my life.

"I can't remember a time when you weren't either on a diet, or worried about your weight," says my sister Suzanne. "Mom always looked trim to me, but I remember her being on *Weight Watchers*. I thought dieting was just what women did."

It was certainly something I needed to do. My sister Debb says I was born "a good eater." When she was a toddler, she bit the leg off a tiny glass deer at our granny's house. The pediatrician advised my mother to make a big bowl of mashed potatoes and to get Debb to eat as much as she could, presumably to cushion the glass piece as it went through her system. She ate about two tablespoons, and I finished the rest.

When other kids were eating peanut butter and jelly or bologna sandwiches in the elementary school cafeteria, I was trying to hide the string-bean salad my mom had brown-bagged for me, her chunky firstborn. I have three sisters and a brother, and I was the only one who was a chubby kid. Back then my eating and weight were a family issue, although today I might have blended in better with all the other overweight kids in the United States. In my preteen years my mother searched for clothes to "slenderize" me, while Debb wore a rubber band for a belt.

Mika told me her family home was junk food free. The same was true of the suburban New York house where I grew up. My sister Melissa recalls, "We were always on a diet in our house. We never had the same snacks as other kids. We never had soda, except on holidays. To this day, my childhood friends remember our house as the one with the empty fridge."

Mom doled out portions of cookies and snack food as treats. She would hide the snacks so none of us could be tempted to sit down and eat a whole bag. I'd go to set the table and discover, tucked in the bottom of the salad bowl, a package of cookies stowed safely out of sight. We didn't have chips unless we were having a party, and we certainly did not eat in front of the TV.

"Good foods and bad foods were clearly defined," says Melissa. "The constant fear of getting fat was drilled into us. Fat was bad, thin was good."

Somehow I didn't get the message, and I managed to keep packing on pounds. There was talk of sending me to "fat camp" for the summer, though that never happened. I was self-conscious about my size, and being the tallest kid in the class didn't help. I was the only twelve-year-old I knew who was on Weight Watchers. My mom cooked and counted calories for my dad and me, and for a while that made a difference.

By high school I had slimmed down, but staying that way through college involved a constant roller coaster of diets. You name it, I tried it. "I never really questioned what you were doing," said Debb about my teen and young adult diet cycles. "It seemed that trying different diets in search of 'the one' was the norm. No one in our circle ever thought to eat less and move more. That was too boring. We just assumed there must be a magic bullet."

I hunted for it, that's for sure.

Remember the Candy Diet from the 1970s? Ayds (pronounced "aids") looked and tasted like chocolates or caramels, but as I found out later, they were appetite suppressants. In the early eighties as the AIDS epidemic broke out, you can imagine what happened to the candy with the similar name. Just as well: the active ingredient was phenylpropanolamine (PPA), which has now been linked to strokes in women.

Still, that one was more fun than the Grapefruit Diet, also known as the Hollywood Diet. It dates back to the 1920s, but became popular again when I was a teen. Lunch and dinner consisted of grapefruit, lean meat, vegetables, and black coffee. The diet came back into vogue yet again in 2004, when a study showed that the enzymes in grapefruit help reduce insulin levels and encourage weight loss (perhaps not coincidentally, the study was sponsored by the Florida Department of Citrus). At 800 calories a day the diet was hard to stick with, and to this day I can't stand to look at grapefruit.

Then there was the Cambridge Diet, which consisted of meal replacement drinks and claimed to provide all the nutrients needed to maintain good health while the dieter lost tremendous amounts of weight. A Cambridge University professor got the credit for that one, and the product sold briskly in the United Kingdom and the United States. The Cambridge Diet worked for a while, but my weight came back on when I started eating real food again. That didn't stop me from trying another liquid diet, Slim-Fast, when I was thirty and hoping to drop a lot of weight before my wedding.

There was always another diet to try, so I kept hopscotching from one to the next. When I went off Slim-Fast I lived on Lean Cuisine. Then there was the Cabbage Soup Diet, with its gallons of cabbage broth, a little coffee, skim milk, and low-fat yogurt. Not surprisingly, the side effects included low energy, mood swings, and sugar cravings.

I can go on and on about my low-cal escapades. How could I forget my bout with the Scarsdale Diet, invented by Dr. Herman Tarnower, whose best-selling diet book was published in 1978? It got another huge sales boost when he was killed two years later by his lover, Jean Harris, headmistress of the Madeira School, Mika's high school alma mater. (When she applied to the school for admission, Mika was interviewed by Harris herself. Not long after, Harris was convicted and sent to prison.)

The South Beach Diet and the Zone Diet had a less colorful backstory, but those were on my list of tried-and-failed diets, too.

Starting to see a pattern here? The pounds came off, but not for long, which led to another round of dieting. Every diet seemed to work for a while, but I never changed my eating habits. I never tried to understand the underlying drivers of my ballooning weight. That wasn't something many of the diet books or the TV talk shows emphasized.

"We come from a mindset that suggests diets are temporary tortures we must endure," says Debb. And when we're done, "then we have permission to backslide into old habits, as if we were entitled to a reward for our sacrifice."

———

Eating for comfort was a well-established pattern for me by the time tragedy struck in my life, and I really needed that comfort. Shortly after graduating from college, the death of my longtime boyfriend following a fiery car crash sent me on a binge of eating and drinking that skyrocketed my weight from 140 pounds to nearly 190. I'll never forget the moment Mom and Dad walked into my newsroom in upstate New York, a three-hour drive from their home. My heart stopped. They took me aside and told me that Mitch had been in a terrible car accident on his way up to see me over the weekend. I had been frantic with worry, not knowing where he was. Even his mother hadn't been able to find him.

Finally the hospital called, and we learned Mitch was in critical condition in the burn unit at a New York City hospital. They had not been able to locate family or friends because most of his possessions in the car had been burned, too. We went to New York and the scene was as horrific as any I hope ever to see in my life. This young man, whom I had loved since he was a boy, was entirely wrapped in bandages. Only his toes were showing, and as I held on to that one part of his body that was unscathed, I prayed, for him and for me. He hung on for a little over a week, until one last brother from his big family was notified and flew home from across the globe. His brother said good-bye and Mitch was gone.

I had just started my TV career and I was living alone. Food was my comfort, and after Mitch's death I kept getting heavier and heavier. It was some time before I was ready to emerge from the darkness of my grief and even think about losing weight.

This time, at my parents' urging and with their encouragement, I turned to the Atkins Diet. Cardiologist Robert C. Atkins described his low-carbohydrate regimen in a series of books, starting with Dr. Atkins' New Diet Revolution in 1972. His approach was controversial, but at one time one in eleven Americans was said to be following the Atkins diet.

It allowed steak, lobster, cheese, and eggs but severely limited carbohydrates. I inhaled food like ham and cheese omelets, burgers (no bun), and nuts. Dr. Atkins contended that his approach switched the body from metabolizing glucose as energy to converting body fat to energy, a process called ketosis that involves controlling the production of insulin in the body.

I remember my first visit with Dr. Atkins. He reviewed my meager breakfast, which typically consisted of toast, coffee, and orange juice, and declared, "That juice is the problem. You've ruined a whole day right there with all that sugar." Mom and Dad picked up the tab for my weekly visits to Atkins' swanky, art-filled Manhattan offices, and for the steaks I sometimes devoured, with the doctor's blessing. I peeled off fifty pounds, and kept them off for a few years. My dad did well on the diet, too.

In the end, the Atkins approach was just one more temporary fix, but dieting in one form or another still remained a habit. I was not much for exercising, unlike Mika, who was fanatical about it. I grew up in the years before Title IX, the federal legislation that required schools to spend equally on sports for men and women. Sports were not built into my school life, and as a kid who was overweight and klutzy, I didn't really learn to play any team sports very well, although I took tennis and swimming lessons.

Women going to a gym to work out? Back then that was virtually unheard of. But I did join an Elaine Powers Figure Salon, an exercise studio designed for women. We donned leotards and tights and danced our way through an early form of aerobics. In those days they still had machines with belts that you put around your hips; I guess we thought that would "jiggle the fat away."

The dancing, combined with some Jane Fonda exercise tapes, kept my weight down for a while. Through my early TV career I managed to maintain a pretty good look. I was never skinny, but with the right camera shots I was attractive enough. In the 1980s, a size 10 was considered fine for a woman on TV. Today, an anchorwoman that large would be considered an elephant.

I moved from my first TV job in Binghamton, New York, where I'd gone to college and started my career, to the Hartford–New Haven TV market. It was a big jump and I loved it. It gave me the chance every day to share the news with our viewers, to tell them stories that would make a difference in their lives. Viewers took me into their homes and their hearts, even sending cards to me at the station when Tom and I got married. They felt like family, and we invited them to our wedding on TV. I am sure they noticed my struggle with weight over the years, but the audience had become my friend—and as Mika has pointed out, friends are sometimes too kind to say what they think.

In my thirties and forties I continued to exercise, joining gyms and even hiring personal trainers, but it wasn't enough. Although I felt better, my weight continued to climb, slowly for a while, then with gathering speed. I would get "too busy" to exercise and fall off that wagon, too.

I kept searching for a permanent weight-loss secret. I had spurts of success with portion-controlled meals from Nutrisystem. Their freeze-dried or frozen foods helped me stay in a size 12 or 14 for a while, until it was time to eat "real food" again. The switch to real-life eating was always my downfall. Counting points, calories, and grams of fat, figuring food exchanges, and every other way of measuring and weighing food made me crazy. I tried Weight Watchers, though I dreaded going to meetings and having people whisper, "That's the gal from the news." I should have gotten past it and said, "Hell, yeah, it is . . . and I am just like you, I need help," but I was too embarrassed.

I'd be vigilant for a while and lose some weight. Then I would hit a plateau and think, Why bother? *Or I'd start sneaking snacks that "didn't count," like a spoonful of peanut butter right out of the jar, or anything that I could eat over the sink. A glass of wine on Saturday night became a cocktail and a glass of wine, and eventually I was having a glass or two every night of the week. I tried to be honest and count the calories allotted for the day or the week, but eventually the counting and the weighing and the vigilance would break down again.*

Luckily for me, my husband was always supportive of my weight-loss efforts. I never suffered from the sabotage syndrome so many women complain about. He wasn't ordering pepperoni pizzas while I was dieting, but when I was willing to indulge, he was, too, and that meant Friday night pizza or Chinese takeout and lots of eating out. I'd indulge, feeling like a normal person for a while. But I never compensated quickly for the extra calories, so I steadily gained weight. Then I'd be back on another strict regimen, trying to drop twenty-five or more pounds.

Over time I went from a size 10 to a 16. Talk about denial.

The only time in my life when I was not obsessed with food was in the mid-1990s, when my doctor prescribed the drug combination fenfluramine-phentermine, commonly known as fen-phen. Losing weight became effortless because I was never hungry. I stopped thinking about food all the time. For the first time in my life I could go to a party without heading to the buffet table. I no longer cleaned my plate at every meal and our dog discovered table scraps for the first time, because there actually were leftovers. I packed a lunch for work, and at the end of the week five of them would be sitting in the newsroom fridge. I had forgotten to eat, something that was once unheard of for me.

I got back to my ideal weight and actually wore a size 10 again. I was elated, and not only because of the serotonin release triggered by the drugs. But as my TV station's consumer reporter used to say, "If a deal seems too good to be true, it probably is." That was definitely the case with fen-phen. A thirty-eight-year-old client at the nail salon I frequented, who had been obese since childhood, started using fen-phen about the same time I did. She got very thin, and then suddenly died. There was no autopsy, but people whispered that fen-phen had killed her.

This made me nervous, but I kept on using it because it felt so good to be thin again. As a TV journalist I even reported on studies suggesting the dangers of fen-phen, but my desire to look good was so strong that I ignored the health risks. I was probably lucky when the matter was taken out of my hands. By the late 1990s, the drug combination had been linked to pulmonary hypertension and heart valve problems and pulled from the market. I decided not to join the class action lawsuits against the manufacturers, but I held my breath for years, fearing that cardiac damage would show up. Thank goodness it never did.

I kept the weight off for a while even without the drug, but as you have probably figured out by now, I gained it all back.

—*uuu*—

For me and just about everyone else who has weight issues, the real trouble is keeping off the pounds after you lose them. I've always felt a kinship with Mark Twain, who once observed, "It's easy to quit smoking. I've done it hundreds of times." The same could be said of me; just substitute the words lose weight *for* smoking. *I can't even begin to calculate how many pounds I have lost and gained over the years.*

When I was forty-nine I set a goal: 50 by 50, meaning I would lose fifty pounds by my fiftieth birthday. At that point I was out of TV news and commuting three hours a day, round trip, to my radio job. My alarm went off at 2:30 a.m. After I had done my radio show, most days I headed to the PBS station in Hartford where I produced and hosted a magazine show. I was tired, but I knew I had to start exercising again if I was going to reach my goal. I joined a gym and lost about twenty pounds. I was on my way to 50 by 50.

Then my health problems began. First came stress fractures in both feet, then a painful neuroma in one foot that led to plantar fasci-

itis and tendonitis. I spent the entire summer in physical therapy. Pain kept me out of the gym, and my weight inched back up. A year later I tripped over my dog (yes, really) and broke my foot and my elbow. Another reason not to go to the gym.

With few other options to consider, I began to think about bariatric surgery. It seemed like an easy answer. Just about everyone who undergoes the surgery loses weight—a lot of it and quickly, too. Bette, a gifted video editor and one of my close friends, had gone through the "lap band" procedure, and I watched how well it worked for her. In gastric banding, a surgeon actually wraps a device around the upper part of the stomach to form a ring. The ring is attached by a tube to an access port left under the skin. The doctor can then control how tight the ring is by inserting saline through the port. So your "new" stomach is smaller, you eat less, and feel full with what seemed to me like teeny amounts of food. Bette lost more than two hundred pounds. Even more importantly, other health problems, known by the scary term comorbidities, cleared up.

Prior to the surgery, Bette had been taking insulin and two oral medications for diabetes, two medications for high blood pressure, and one for her cholesterol. She suffered from swelling so severe that sometimes she could barely keep shoes on her feet. And because she had developed sleep apnea, a dangerous condition closely linked to overweight, she was tethered at night to a continuous positive airway pressure (CPAP) machine to help her breathe.

After surgery Bette needed none of that. She was off all her medications, worked out almost daily at a gym, started riding a motorcycle, and trained to be an emergency medical technician. She even posed nude for an art class. It was obvious the weight loss had transformed her life, and I suspect it may have even saved it.

But like most medical procedures, bariatric surgery has its down-

sides, and I saw some of those up close with Bette. Vomiting, nausea, nighttime acid reflux, and other postoperative complications can be enduring problems. Bette also had a significant amount of loose skin, and considered extensive plastic surgery to get rid of it.

Still, bariatric surgery was tempting. There are a number of possible approaches, but as I did my research, I was not entirely surprised to learn that none of them are the perfect fix they appear to be. Never mind the TV stars you see showing off their sexy new bodies after bariatric surgery. It is definitely not that simple.

The procedure does change your life, but some of the long-term implications are daunting. I wasn't sure I could live permanently on a diet that counts a half cup of food as a full meal, requires that you chew your food to the consistency of a fine paste, and advises you not to eat food and drink liquids at the same time.

I was also concerned about one common and often permanent side effect of "gastric bypass," which is a type of bariatric surgery that involves disconnecting the stomach from the small intestine and connecting it to the large intestine instead. The side effect, called dumping syndrome, *happens when the undigested contents of the stomach move too rapidly into the small bowel. When people who have had the surgery eat sweets, dairy, fats, or carbohydrates they sometimes get very ill with symptoms that can include weakness, feeling faint, nausea, sweating, cramping, and diarrhea.*

I had watched two other friends struggle with the aftermath of bariatric surgery. One woman about my age had a procedure called vertical sleeve gastrectomy. *Her surgeon removed 85 percent of her stomach. She chose that procedure because it avoids some of the side effects and weight regain that can accompany gastric bypass. Still, a full meal for her is about three ounces of food, and she must be constantly vigilant about what she eats. The other friend is much younger, barely out of her teenage years, and she spent weeks in a hospital and months in recovery after complications from her gastric bypass.*

Despite all that, both women considered the procedure to be a life saver. But they were also substantially heavier than I am. With a BMI of 38, I was just below the level that officially qualified for the surgery, though I'm pretty sure I could have persuaded a doctor to take me on as a patient.

Another downside was the cost. The lap band procedure can cost between $8,000 and $30,000. My insurance company would have paid for it if I had a BMI of 40 or above, or a BMI of 35 coupled with a comorbidity, such as diabetes. Thankfully, I had no comorbid conditions.

All the medical literature says the surgery is to be used only as a last resort. It might have been worth paying for it out of pocket if it was truly my only option, but I couldn't convince myself of that, despite my long and checkered career as a dieter. Wouldn't it really be better to improve my eating habits and exercise more? Reluctantly, I ruled out surgery. There had to be another way.

—⌇⌇⌇—

At the time Mika hit me over the head about my weight, I was in deep denial about how dire my situation was. I was in my mid-fifties and weighed 250 pounds. There, I said it. 250 pounds. I can hardly breathe just writing down that number on the page. It is so shocking, even to me. I weighed more than some NFL players.

At the time Mika hit me over the head about my weight, I was in deep denial about how dire my situ-

***ation was. I was in my mid-fifties and weighed 250 pounds.*—Diane**

How did this happen? I look in the mirror and I cannot believe what I see. I was never skinny, but at size 10, I was once described by a TV critic as "comely." Now I am pushing a size 20*? My heart is pounding as I read and reread this line, but I'll say it again: 250 pounds.*

"You're fat," Mika said. I was.

I began to craft a program that I hope will bring long-term permanent change. I'm done with promises of a quick fix, and I know from experience that restricting what I eat is not enough. After years of yo-yo dieting, I know firsthand that people who don't exercise lose muscle and fat while dieting, but when they rebound, they gain back the fat.

The first thing I needed to do was to get off the couch and into the gym. But with all my pains, aches, and general loss of fitness, I was nervous about getting injured. Those stress fractures in my feet, which developed after the ambitious weight-loss program I had started several years earlier, eventually led to a raft of related orthopedic problems. For several years I had been in and out of physical therapy. I couldn't afford to go through all of that again.

I asked my doctor and my physical therapist how to transition from physical therapy into the gym without injury, but neither had a solid recommendation. I'd worked with trainers on and off with some success, but this time I needed someone who could also address the myriad medical issues I was developing. I looked at sev-

eral hospital-sponsored programs, but most were targeted at cardiac patients.

The more I looked, the less I was convinced I could find a trainer and a gym that could really help me. I knew I couldn't afford another injury, and besides, in my current condition I was less than enthusiastic about being surrounded by Skinny Minnies. Then two very caring friends came to me with a suggestion (you might even call it an intervention). They were getting great results with a trainer who had a radically new approach and a rare ability to motivate clients and inspire change.

My friend Anna is fit and athletic, but she'd had to undergo knee surgery. She said this trainer had helped her to heal, and to take her workouts to a new level. The other friend is a TV weatherman whose weight had climbed to over three hundred pounds. Joe was a longtime colleague, and I knew he had struggled with his weight for years. He was turning fifty, and had recently lost eighty pounds and maintained the loss. He said he was in better shape than he had been in his days playing college football. The trainer, he told me, counseled him on nutrition and "gets inside your head."

At their urging, I looked into Akua Ba Fitness, a one-on-one training center in West Hartford operated by D'Mario Sowah. I needed someone special. My fear of being injured again, coupled with my embarrassment about my size, called for someone who could go above and beyond the usual requirements. It was a tough combination to deal with, but I was lucky enough to meet someone who could. D'Mario is a master trainer who is experienced and well versed in fitness and anatomy. The small size of his studio also meant I would have some privacy—definitely a plus.

In terms of life circumstances, D'Mario and I are polar opposites. He is a young African American born in Ghana, plucked from *an orphanage and forced into slavery as a child soldier. As we worked out together, I slowly learned his extraordinary life story, including his escape that led him to America. The way he rebuilt his life is incredibly uplifting.*

D'Mario's regimen involves healthy eating and a training method that foregoes most exercise equipment, relying instead on using your own body weight as the resistance in your workout. At our first meeting he analyzed my fitness level (virtually nonexistent) and talked to me about my goals and my failure to lose weight over the last fifteen years. My tears flowed (again), and in spite of our differences I sensed the inner spirit of this man, his nurturing soul. About my weight and my awful physical condition, D'Mario simply said, "Lay down that burden; that burden is mine to carry now."

About my weight and my awful physical condition, D'Mario simply said, "Lay down that burden; that burden is mine to carry now."—Diane

No one had ever referred to my weight like that before; as a burden I had been carrying. And yet of course it was. I had felt so much shame because I had not been able to rid myself of it. I felt like a failure after all the false starts, all the dashed hopes of recent years.

Through my career I had been seen as a winner: popular, talented, and able to reinvent myself every time a curve ball was thrown my way. When I was downsized from my position as a news anchor, I became a morning talk show host at the biggest radio station in the state, and landed a contract to produce and host programs at the PBS network in Connecticut. I turned my TV work into six successful books.

But at the age of fifty, after I was downsized from the radio job and had my PBS work outsourced after ten successful years, I was shaken. And now I couldn't even control my own body. I was fat and feeling miserable.

It wasn't easy for me to let go of the sunny personality I showed the world, but D'Mario let me see that I could, at least in the privacy of our training sessions. "I want you to let go of the pain and just believe," he said. "That's hard, but I want to help you see that this is just a stage of your life, and there is a lot more ahead for you."

So I started Mika's challenge with new optimism. Little did I know that a major health crisis would derail my plan, and that I would spend months getting back on track. This journey was going to be a bumpy ride.

CHAPTER FOUR

FAT: WHOSE FAULT?

My story, with Mayor Michael Bloomberg,
Governor Chris Christie, Rebecca Puhl,
Senator Claire McCaskill, Dr. David Katz,
David Kirchhoff, Frank Bruni, Gayle King,
Dr. Emily Senay, Lisa Powell, Dr. Ezekiel Emanuel,
Ashley Gearhardt, Michael Prager, Joe Scarborough,
Brian Stelter, Dr. Robert Lustig, Kimber Stanhope,
Lewis Cantley

Not long ago on *Morning Joe*, New York City mayor Michael Bloomberg made a startling statement. "This year more people in the world will die of the complications of overweight than from starvation."

Have we all really turned into gluttons? Are we all poorly disciplined and lacking character? It just can't be that our nation's collective weight problem is entirely our fault as individuals. With so many Americans overweight, something else must be going on. Each of us may have our own challenges, but it is the nation that has an obesity crisis. As New Jersey Governor Chris Christie said, it is ignorant "to believe that being overweight is merely a function of willpower."

And yet that is just what we tend to think, says Yale researcher Rebecca Puhl. "The prevailing perception in our culture is that obesity is an issue of lack of willpower, lack of discipline, or personal responsibility." Each one of us tends to think we are struggling alone.

I'm convinced that a lot more is involved. To get to the root of the problem, we need to look hard in many directions. At the highly processed food that is so readily available. At the systems we have structured to make food that is laden with fat, sugar, and salt so much cheaper than wholesome foods. At the vending machines in school, hospital, and employee cafeterias where chips, candy, and soda are the only things available. At the limits of the labeling requirements we impose on food in stores and restaurants. At the look we consider healthy and beautiful, especially in our young girls. At how we talk about weight with one another.

I can go on and on about the sources of the problem, because we have created a hydra-headed monster here. We've surrounded ourselves with unhealthy foods that we just can't stop eating.

Here is one shocking example: students consume almost 400 billion junk food calories at school every year according to *Still Too Fat to Fight*, a 2012 report by Mission: Readiness.[1] That's equal to almost 2 billion candy bars. (The report also notes that the weight of those candy bars is considerably more than the weight of the *Midway*, the longest-serving aircraft carrier in the US Navy.)

At the same time, as few as 4 percent of high school students have the opportunity to take a daily gym class. We're setting them up to become fat.

Yes, of course we all need to take personal responsibility, but those kinds of statistics suggest we should be thinking differently about what that really means. It's not just that we are responsible for getting our own weight under control, although that's part of the solution. But we also need to think about the role each of us can play in initiating conversations that can change the whole society.

"We can control our health care costs, we can control our national debt and our deficit if everybody in America would recognize obesity as the public health hazard that it has become," declares Senator Claire McCaskill.

> **We can control our health care costs, we can control our national debt and our deficit if everybody in America would recognize obesity as the public health hazard that it has become.**
> **—*Senator Claire McCaskill***

To understand how we got here, let's take a look at evolution and human biology.

"The truth is, we are the first generation, or the second, where getting fat is the path of least resistance," says David Katz, MD, director of the Yale Prevention Research Center and editor of the medical journal *Childhood Obesity*. "Throughout most of human history, people were struggling to get enough to eat." For most Americans, that struggle is a thing of the past. "If you look at the food supply of the United States today versus, say, 1970, we have about five hundred to six hundred additional calories available per capita per day now than we did then," explains David Kirchhoff, CEO of Weight Watchers. "Most of those new foods are coming with added sugars and fats, otherwise known as heavily processed foods and known in some quarters as junk food."

Our biology makes it hard to say no to junk food. We're hardwired to go after the concentrated energy in high-calorie fats and sweets. Just look at me: I know that empty calories are the quickest route to unwanted pounds, and that's the last thing I want. I know I'll have to make up for an extra snack with an extra run. I've learned these lessons the hard way, and I've learned them over and over again. Yet what I know flies out the window when I see that bag of chips or that pint of ice cream; it's as if my body is overriding my logic. There are days when I struggle not to pick up the fork.

Same thing with Diane. She loses the battle more often than I do, yet she's got more drive than most people I know. Her problem is not that she lacks discipline.

What's really going on here?

"We're simply not genetically programmed to refuse calories when they're within arm's reach." That's what Thomas Farley, New York City's health commissioner, told *New York Times* columnist Frank Bruni. Bruni makes the case that America's obesity crisis is partially the result of its prosperity and economic dominance. "Over the last century," he writes, "we became expert at the mass production of crops like corn, soybeans and wheat—a positive development, for the most part."[2]

The less positive element in that equation is that America also became efficient at "processing those crops into salty, sweet, fatty, cheap, and addictive seductions," Bruni explains. "Densely caloric and all-too-convenient food now envelops us, and many of us do what we're chromosomally hardwired to, thanks to millenniums of feast-and-famine cycles. We devour it."

Densely caloric and all-too-convenient food now envelops us.—*Frank Bruni*

Soda and sugary drinks are one of the worst culprits, providing the single largest source of calories in the American diet. We're drinking twice as much of them as we did forty years ago. For many Americans, it's all feast and no famine. We no longer need those stores of energy to keep us going through the lean times. Instead, the extra calories turn into fat.

"We are products of our times," says Yale's David Katz. "Human character hasn't changed, personal responsibility hasn't changed, but the world has changed, and it's a very obesigenic world."

⁓⁓⁓

One feature of that world is that food is everywhere, available 24/7, and marketed to the tune of some $36 billion per year. Yale's Rudd Center reports that the fast food industry alone spends $4 billion in advertising yearly, much of it aimed at children.[3] By comparison, for every dollar the industry spends pushing fast food, the US Department of Agriculture spends about one-tenth of a penny encouraging people to eat their vegetables.

When there's a downturn in the economy, those marketing dollars flow even more freely, and the stock prices of fast food companies often rise as they roll out offers like "dollar menus" and consumers perceive fast food meals as bargains. There is definitely a payoff in the corporate bottom line. Marketing dollars spent translates into food eaten. One survey by the Rudd

Center showed that the week before it was conducted, 84 percent of parents had taken their child to a fast food restaurant.[4]

I remember watching fast food ads when I was a kid, and I clearly remember that they sparked cravings in me. And I am certainly not the only one to hear the food marketers' siren calls. My friend Gayle King, who co-hosts *CBS This Morning*, says she has never stopped being motivated by commercials. "You're talking to somebody who saw a McRib commercial and left the house in the rain," Gayle chuckles. "I put on some boots and took an umbrella because the McRib sandwich was a limited-time offer! So I went to McDonald's in the rain, though the whole time I'm saying to myself, 'Turn around. Turn around. Turn around.'"

Supermarkets jump into the game, too, deliberately placing candy bars, sweet snacks, and sugary cereals where children will see them. "In most places, the bad food is about eye level of where the kids are," points out Dr. Emily Senay, a *Morning Joe* regular who teaches in the Department of Preventive Health at Mount Sinai School of Medicine and is the medical correspondent for the PBS show *Need to Know*. "The candy, the chips, all that stuff is low enough in the store where they can easily see it. If you have little kids, it makes going out on a simple excursion a battle. The world we live in conspires against us when it comes to healthy eating."

Even if you avoid fast food chains and choose healthy foods in the market, eating out a lot is also asking for trouble because serving sizes in most restaurants have grown so dramatically in this country. The Centers for Disease Control and Prevention (CDC) estimates that restaurant portion sizes are more than four times larger now than they were in the 1950s.

If portion sizes had increased overnight, says Lisa Powell, director of Nutrition at Canyon Ranch Health Resort in Tucson, Arizona, "people would be horrified. But it was just a little here, a little there, and our eyes got used to it and our stomachs got used to it. It makes me fear for people who are under thirty years old because it means they've never seen normal portions modeled."

—*uun*—

The world that Dr. Katz calls "obesigenic" is also a place where takeout and packaged foods dominate, and healthy home cooking has become increasingly rare. A report led by Harvard University economists says that in the 1960s, "the bulk of food preparation was done by families that cooked their own food and ate it at home. Since then there has been a revolution in the mass preparation of food that is roughly comparable to the mass production revolution in manufactured goods that happened a century ago."[5]

In 1965, a married woman who didn't work outside the home spent over two hours a day cooking meals and cleaning up afterward. By 1995, that same woman spent less than half that time in the kitchen. As we moved into the twenty-first century, those numbers fell even further. We spend less and less time preparing meals at home, and people eat more and more mass-produced foods. Cooking from scratch seems to have become a hobby for a small group of people and a chore that the rest of us no longer bother with.

"My grandmother's full-time job, basically, was to feed a big family, and she worked from morning till night," says Canyon

Ranch's Lisa Powell. "In the sixties, women were beginning to enter the workforce, and the notion of convenience foods became popular. As our society changed, the environment was ripe for packaged and processed foods, which saved time. Today, you get your food out of a box or a can, you don't have to think about it, you don't have to mess with it, and you don't have to touch it."

The less frequently we cook, the more we rely on mass-manufactured foods that are quick and easy to prepare. Most people aren't giving much thought to what's packed into them, but Powell certainly is. "Packaged food is high in salt, high in sugar, high in fat—all of those basic, primordial food preferences that people have. Seeking out salt, fat, and sugar ensured survival in previous eras, and we still have that same tendency." The more we consume highly processed foods, she says, "the more our preferences have been directed that way, and we've lost the appreciation for fresh and whole food. The only thing that resonates with people is flavor and the intensity of flavor."

Along with passing up healthier foods for convenience, we have changed some of our basic customs. We no longer expect to eat three meals a day, sitting at a table with our families. In a family dinner setting, people can be more mindful of what they are eating and how much they are consuming. When meals are more "grab and go," we end up doing a lot more grazing and snacking.

"We don't take time to eat," said Lisa Powell. "We stuff in a sandwich at our desk and think we had lunch. We've lost that connection; we've just lost contact with the whole experience of eating. As a result, I think we're not satisfied, so we're looking for more and more and more and more."

We've just lost contact with the whole experience of eating. As a result, I think we're not satisfied, so we're looking for more and more and more and more.—*Lisa Powell*

Then there's the fact that social mores in America encourage eating just about everywhere. "If you go to Japan, it's sort of socially prohibited to eat on the street," says Ezekiel Emanuel, MD, a former White House advisor on health and chair of the Department of Medical Ethics and Health Policy at the University of Pennsylvania. Zeke is also a *Morning Joe* regular. "People just don't do it. It's very different in America."

Price also plays a role. The fact is that eating nutritious food is more expensive than the alternative. "Compared to things like fresh fruits and vegetables, processed foods have a decreased price per calorie, and the economists will tell you that has a role," Emanuel acknowledges.

On top of that, our lives no longer require much physical activity. The kind of hard labor we used to do has been largely replaced by machines. We no longer walk to work; we drive. We have to deliberately seek opportunities to burn off calories because they are no longer built into everyday life, as they were for earlier generations. Put that together with today's food environment and we begin to understand why we've gotten fat.

"Everything about modern living that makes it modern is obesigenic," says Katz. "The problem is a flood of highly processed, hyperpalatable, energy-dense, nutrient-diluted, glow-in-the-dark, bet-you-can't-eat-just-one kind of foods" coupled with "wave after wave of technological advances giving us devices to do all the things muscles used to do."

The problem is a flood of highly processed, hyper-palatable, energy-dense, nutrient-diluted, glow-in-the-dark, bet-you-can't-eat-just-one kind of foods.
                                                    —*David Katz*

That pretty much sums up why the American obesity crisis started about forty years ago. David Kirchhoff of Weight Watchers calls it "a perfect storm of overeating and under-exercising."

———*᠊ᴍᴍ*᠊———

If my theory that some of us are addicted to unhealthy foods is confirmed by science, we'll be able to understand a lot more about why we eat when we don't want to. Ashley Gearhardt, PhD, a faculty member in the Department of Clinical Psychology at the University of Michigan, is a research pioneer in that area. When, as a graduate student at Yale University, she first began examining the possibility that food could be addictive, the very idea was mocked. Now, people are looking a lot more closely at the science that could explain food addiction, and her work is considered groundbreaking.

Although we still need to understand the biology better, it is no longer fringe thinking to suggest that foods "jacked up in their level of sugar, fat, and salt are addictive to some people," says Gearhardt. "I think one reason that people don't take food addiction seriously is because we all need food to survive. But in looking at the obesity epidemic, you realize that it's a certain type of food that shows this addictive potential."

The villain is no surprise: the food we call *ultraprocessed*, or highly palatable. Another term for it is *junk food*. It contains ingredients in quantities that are simply not natural to the body.

Gearhardt's research is built on well-accepted principles of addiction. As she explains it, the addictive potential of any substance is based on two factors: the speed of its absorption into the body and the level of activation in the brain's reward system. "If you look at a food that's naturally occurring, like a banana, it has a decent amount of sugar in it, but it comes naturally packaged in a way that is high in fiber and high in other antioxidants that slow down the absorption of the sugar into our bloodstream," she explains.

Now, let's compare that to a handful of jellybeans. There is more sugar in the candy, but more significantly, that sugar gets into the bloodstream a lot faster because it has no fiber or antioxidants. This means our response to the rewards in those jellybeans is a lot stronger than our response to the rewards in the banana—and that's what can make a food addictive.

"There are foods that are naturally elevated in sugar, like fruits, and there are foods that are naturally elevated in fat, like nuts and meats, but there are very, very few foods that are naturally elevated in both sugar and fat," notes Gearhardt. "Just by combining sugar and fat, we're creating a food that is abnormally rewarding." That's why we crave it. "So even though you know it's causing you massive health issues and mental health concerns, you feel compelled to keep consuming it and really struggle to stop," she says.

Sounds a lot like a drug addict, doesn't it?

Besides fat, sugar, and salt, Gearhardt says other additives in foods, such as caffeine, have properties that make them potentially addictive. And caffeine sometimes shows up in places that the average consumer wouldn't expect—like candy and chips. "If you are consuming caffeine in these products, you're going to crave it a little more and feel a little more withdrawal when you stop eating it," she says. Gearhardt's research shows that a person eventually needs more of the processed food to get the same pleasurable response, another classic signal of addiction. In other words, if one handful of M&Ms is good, the whole package is better.

Zeke Emanuel is a little less certain that processed foods are actually addictive, but he does think the theory needs further study. "It's being explored, how the brain becomes habituated to certain things and not others," he responds. "For anyone to definitively say, 'Yes, there's an addiction pathway there that these manufactured foods plug into'—I think it's just too early in the research. But it's very interesting."

Echoing Governor Christie, he added, "This is not simply a matter of willpower."

Michael Prager is one man who is persuaded that food can be addictive. Prager, who has tipped the scales at 365 pounds, told Diane and me that he once felt totally out of control around food. Now he calls himself a recovering food addict. As a newspaper editor on the *Hartford Courant*, Michael worked the night shift. On his short commute home, he would sometimes get off the highway at an exit that has a Wendy's, Burger King, and McDonald's, side by side by side.

"One time I hit 'em all, the fast food triple play," he told us. "I went through the drive-thru at the first place. I pulled over so I could eat in secret, although I'm fully aware that you can see through the windows of cars. Then I went next door to the next one. I bought another entire meal—soda, fries, sandwich—pulled over, ate it, and then I went to the next one and did the same thing. Three of them at one time. I was trying to get back at people who I had decided had wronged me in some way, as if I could hurt them by doing this."

His bad behavior didn't end there.

"At my worst, you could find me lying on the floor of my living room at three in the morning," Michael continues. "The reason I'm not sitting up anymore is I've had too much food, and it's too painful to be sitting up. And lying down made it possible to get more food in." That was important, he says, because "I was more into volume than I was into any particular substance. I didn't discriminate. I would go to a convenience store after work and get a quart of milk and a box of cereal and a loaf of bread and a jar of peanut butter and a jar of jelly. My goal was to have enough food to get me through the night so that I didn't have to get up at four in the morning to go out and get more.

"At work, I would try to figure out how many times I could go to the vending machine without people noticing. I was over three hundred pounds. People know that I'm an overeater, so who was I kidding? I would go to the vending machine and buy three things and go in the bathroom and eat one of them and then bring one back, and that would be the one that everybody could see. And then I'd have another one that I'd keep in my pocket and try to sneak."

Michael doesn't behave like that anymore, as he explains in his memoir, *Fat Boy, Thin Man*. Today, he follows a food plan that involves weighing and measuring most everything that goes in his mouth. He now weighs 210 pounds, a weight he has maintained for more than twenty years. How did he get there? A big part was in-patient treatment: exactly what a drug addict or an alcoholic needs to confront substance abuse.

Today Michael is a motivational speaker, talking about an addiction he feels was created and nurtured by the "Big Food" makers. "Studies have documented a biochemical sensitivity to hyperpalatable foods, usually processed foods, that promote the phenomenon of cravings and cause people to act unreasonably and irrationally with food, trying to solve other problems," he explains. "If you take out the word *food* and you put in *alcohol* or you put in *cocaine*, the concept of addiction is not controversial."

—*mm*—

Michael's story and his behavior as a food junkie is all too real to me. If we had a medical diagnosis called *food addict*, I'm convinced I would qualify. Most people assume that all food addicts are fat, but I'm here to tell you they are not. Just because I have a healthy body weight doesn't necessarily mean I have a healthy relationship with food.

Most people don't know that I still fight my cravings for "bad food" every day. Even my *Morning Joe* partner, Joe Scarborough, thought I was a highly controlled eater—overly controlled, I think he would say. Joe and my executive producer, Chris Licht, were always pushing me to eat more when we were out on the road together. They thought my diet was far too restrictive, and they were very concerned about me.

And then they became witnesses to a breakdown in my highly disciplined diet. It happened in a big way on one of our road trips, and became an inside joke on *Morning Joe*, although it wasn't all that funny to me. Joe told the story to Diane when she interviewed him.

"We were in Dallas at a Bob Schieffer journalism symposium at Texas Christian University, and we had been going from five in the morning to about ten-thirty at night. We had not had time for dinner, so our producer Louis ordered Mexican food for us to take in the car on our way to the airport.

"I swear to God, I heard in the backseat of the Suburban what sounded like raccoons going through the ten plates of Mexican enchiladas. Mika had devoured a meal that was intended for, like, four or five people. She'd eaten the entire thing and she had this sauce all over her face and going down the front of her shirt.

"I said, 'What in the hell are you doing?'

"And she snapped out of her trance and said, 'Oh, my god. Oh, my god.'"

Joe said that was the first time he truly realized just how extreme a battle I sometimes fought with food.

Ashley Gearhardt's interest in food addiction is rooted in part in her own weakness for some of these foods. She recalls how, during a time crunch, she stopped at a vending machine in the basement of the psychology department and bought an ancient package of Oreos. She said the cookies tasted like cardboard, but that didn't stop her from eating every one.

"I ate the whole package because my body's responding to

this jolt of sugar, jolt of fat that I'm getting, even though it really didn't taste that great," she recalls. "Most foods have been changed and altered in a way that really resembles how we've created drugs of abuse."

Gearhardt developed the Yale Food Addiction Scale to identify people who are most likely to show a dependency on high-fat, high-sugar foods. The scale evaluates classic signs of addiction, such as tolerance and consumption, by asking people to indicate how frequently they engage in certain behaviors, such as these:

- I find that when I start eating certain foods, I end up eating much more than planned.
- I find myself continuing to consume certain foods even though I am no longer hungry.
- I eat to the point where I feel physically ill.
- Over time, I have found that I need to eat more and more to get the feeling I want, such as reduced negative emotions or increased pleasure.

She offered me a compelling portrait of the food addict. "You need more and more of the substance to get the same effect that you once did. You used to eat a couple of cookies, and that was enough for you. Now you find yourself eating the whole pack and wanting more."

Like drug addicts, food addicts also show signs of withdrawal, like anxiety, agitation, headaches, and disrupted sleep, when they try to cut down or stop eating addictive food. Another similarity is that they often know their behavior is causing them physical and emotional problems, and hurting their personal relationships, but they find themselves unable to change it.

Food addicts also devote considerable time to the pursuit of food. "There's a lot of time spent purchasing the substance, using the substance, recovering from the effects of the substance," Gearhardt told me. "So rather than going out and socializing or going on a walk, your life starts to revolve around the substance."

It may sound a lot like a cocaine addiction or alcoholism, but we're talking here about the "ultraprocessed" foods available to us at every turn.

New York Times reporter Brian Stelter is someone else who relates personally to the concept of food addiction. His cravings lingered long after he lost that hundred pounds. "I increasingly felt it myself when I would pass by McDonald's or Burger King or Cinnabon, and I never felt that tug walking by the grocery store where there were fresh fruits and vegetables."

It's a tug he came to resent. "Let's assume that there's some element of weakness there. Maybe it's 25 percent, 50 percent, 75 percent, but I also assume there's some piece of it that's addicting. I began to actually resent it. I would still eat at McDonald's—I love their salads. But I didn't like the tug I felt toward the other food when I was there. I wish I hadn't ever tried it.

"It's funny to say those words because it sounds like a drug. I felt it even more after I'd lost the weight. I don't know if that's because my body became so used to whatever chemicals and additives are in fast food. I guess that my body is missing and craving those substances, whatever they are.

"That's what's so frustrating about this moment in the culture: that there's so much we don't know about what this food does to us."

———

Most overweight people are not food addicts, so dealing with food addiction won't address the entire obesity challenge, but it's certainly part of it. Researcher Ashley Gearhardt studied a population of people who had been diagnosed with disordered eating and found that about half of disordered eating individuals met the addiction threshold. Around 10 percent of college students met the threshold.[6]

But the more we learn about our response to highly processed foods, the more likely it seems that there's something biochemical going on in our bodies. You don't have to be an addict to find your determination breaking down in the face of foods rich in sugar, fat, and salt. You just have to be pulled in by their sensory power.

Lisa Powell calls some of our food "anti-nourishing, if not downright toxic." We're being fed, she says, but we're not being nourished. "And I think that plays a huge role, both physically and psychologically. I think you don't reach that sense of satiety. It has nothing to do with how many calories are in the foods you ate, it has to do with the experience of eating, with the flavor and the roundedness of the experience that we've lost. It's all this intense flavor that just goes in a hurry and we aren't mindful."

In his book *The End of Overeating,* former FDA (US Food and Drug Administration) commissioner David A. Kessler, MD, hearkens back to the comparison between a banana and candy. A handful of M&Ms, he says, has what the food industry calls "better mouth feel. You have to chew less, and they do just 'melt in your mouth.'" That means the sugar and fat hit your system faster and set off a pleasurable reaction. Add to that the constant barrage of advertising and marketing urging you to go out and buy these foods and their ready availability—a combination that Kessler dubs a "food carnival"—and weight gain is the entirely predictable outcome.

"If I give you a pack of sugar, and I say, 'Go have a good time,' you're going to look at me and say, 'What are you talking about?' Now I add to that fat and temperature and texture and mouth feel and color, and I'm going to put it on every corner, and I'm going to say you can do it with your friends, you can do it at the end of the day when you want to relax. Besides making food more irresistible, we made it socially acceptable to eat at any time. What did we expect to happen?"

David Kirchhoff of Weight Watchers describes the effect in a darker way, not as a carnival but as "the equivalent of waterboarding people with food, where eventually you'll break down and you'll start eating." Like so many other people involved in the struggle to bring America's weight down, Kirchhoff fought his own battle, taking nine years to lose forty-five pounds and keep them off.

He writes about brain research in his book *Weight Loss Boss,* and when we interviewed him, he described what happens to many of us at the sight of one of our favorite foods. "A functional MRI can show your brain lighting up like a Christmas tree." The higher functions of the brain may stay in control initially, "telling you *not* to eat whatever the trigger food is—ice cream, chocolate, whatever might be the case. You can avoid that food for a period of time, but then something called *decision fatigue* sets in, and eventually you break down and you'll start to eat it."

When we put this biochemical response together with the food industry's drive to sell its products, the real problems set in. If eating high-fat, high-sugar food prompts people to eat more and more of it, that's what the industry is going to manufacture.

"If you bathe taste buds all the time in excesses of sugar and salt, which is what the typical American diet does, people tend to like products with lots of sugar and lots of salt, and the wrong kinds of fat, and artificial flavorings," explains Yale's David Katz. "Then, if you ask food companies to make products that are much lower in sugar and salt, those products do very badly. Nobody buys them. And then the food companies say, 'Hey, we tried, but we're not going to go out of business to make the public health types happy, so forget about it.' And we get stuck there."

I asked Zeke Emanuel whether he thought food companies were manipulating consumers by creating foods we can't resist. He answered me cautiously. "As an ethicist I'm very careful about the words I use and try to be careful about *manipulation*; it tends to be one of the squishier words. But I would say they *adjust, modify, test,* and *reformulate* the products to increase their palatability," he said. "After all, they want to increase sales. That's how they make their money. They're trying to make us happy with what they're giving us."

—*mm*—

Sugar is a particularly significant culprit in the obesity epidemic, and it is everywhere in the food supply. Some experts say that recommendations to eat a low-fat diet fostered the problem. In the late 1970s, the US Department of Agriculture, the American Medical Association, and the American Heart Association began urging people to reduce their fat intake. Countless Americans heard that message and in many cases began replacing fats with carbs; but instead of getting those carbs primarily from whole grains, fruits, and vegetables, they upped their consumption of bread, pasta, and potatoes.

At the same time, food companies began tinkering with their recipes, according to Robert Lustig, MD, a pediatric endocrinologist at the University of California, San Francisco Benioff Children's Hospital "The food industry was remanded to change its processes. It was basically told 'we have to go low fat,'" says Lustig, who also directs the university's Weight Assessment for Teen and Child Health program. "The problem is that low-fat food tasted like cardboard and the food industry knew that."

To compensate for the loss of flavor, the industry began replacing fat with carbohydrate, especially sugar. And the cheapest sugar available was high-fructose corn syrup, which it now uses in vast amounts. Not only is high-fructose corn syrup cheap, it helps foods last longer on supermarket shelves. "What happened was the 'Great Substitution,'" says Lustig.

"Which is worse for you, the fat or the carbohydrate?" he asks. "When you compare, on balance, the answer is that carbohydrate is worse, because the carbohydrate drives insulin, and insulin drives metabolic disease." Not only do sugars contribute to the obesity epidemic because of their calories, but Lustig is even more concerned about their direct health impact. "Sugar is the factor that takes you from obesity to metabolic syndrome." Metabolic syndrome, which is strongly connected with obesity, is a risk factor for type 2 diabetes, high blood pressure, cholesterol problems, heart disease, and fatty liver disease. And Lustig cautions, "There are implications for cancer and dementia, as well."

> **Sugar is the factor that takes you from obesity to metabolic syndrome.—*Robert Lustig***

No wonder he has labeled sugar "toxic" and is heading a movement against it.

Some people seem to be listening. Lustig's ninety-minute lecture "Sugar: The Bitter Truth" has been viewed more than 3 million times on You Tube since it was posted in July 2009. Listening, perhaps, but not yet acting on the information. It is shocking to me that Americans now consume an average of twenty-two teaspoons of sugar a day. That's 450 calories right there. Compare that to American Heart Association recommendations that men consume no more than nine teaspoons a day and women no more than six teaspoons, amounts that Dr. Lustig says are reasonable, and probably safe.

Why is sugar so bad for us?

In limited quantities, our bodies can handle it, explains Dr. Lustig. Take fructose. Traditionally, it was found mostly in fruit and honey. We can metabolize a certain amount of it, especially if it contains fiber, which delays its absorption in the intestine, and gives the liver a chance to spread out the time it takes to metabolize the food. Exercise also helps, because it speeds up energy metabolism within the liver, allowing the fructose to be turned into energy rather than liver fat. But the much wider use of high-fructose corn syrup puts our health at risk.

"If you overwhelm your liver's capacity to metabolize fructose, then it's a poison," Lustig warns. "A calorie is a calorie in terms of the number of pounds of weight you put on. But that doesn't mean that a calorie is a calorie in terms of the metabolic consequences. If you put those calories in your subcutaneous fat, you just get fat. If you put those calories in your visceral fat or in your muscle or in your liver, then not only are you going to get fat, but you're going to get sick, too."

Studies of how sugary drinks affect the body, conducted by Kimber Stanhope, a nutritional biologist at the University of California–Davis, suggest that Lustig's fears are justified. Her subjects were young, healthy people in a hospital setting where it was possible to measure every calorie they consumed. Within two weeks, those who consumed drinks sweetened with high-fructose corn syrup had higher levels of LDL cholesterol in their blood and other risk factors for heart disease, while the subjects who consumed drinks sweetened with glucose did not. LDL cholesterol, also known as the "bad" cholesterol, collects in the walls of blood vessels, causing blockages and increasing the risk for a heart attack from a sudden blood clot in a compromised artery.

Stanhope explains that all fructose and glucose molecules get delivered directly from the digestive system to the liver. Most of the glucose molecules bypass the liver, because glucose use by the liver is controlled by an enzyme which shuts down when the liver does not need energy. (Glucose, a simple sugar that the body makes when it digests carbohydrates, provides our primary source of fuel.) Therefore, most of the glucose in the drinks sweetened with glucose ended up being used by muscle, brain, and body fat for energy. In contrast, most of the fructose in the drinks sweetened with fructose ended up in the liver. That's because, says Stanhope, "the enzyme that controls fructose use by the liver never shuts down. It efficiently starts processing all the available fructose molecules, which allows the liver to keep bringing more fructose molecules in. The liver has to do something with all this fructose, so it starts turning some of it into fat for later use. Some of this fat gets sent out in the blood where it increases risk factors for cardiovascular disease."

Lewis Cantley, a Harvard professor and head of the Cancer Center at Beth Israel Deaconess Medical Center in Boston, is another scientist very worried about sugar, especially its potential link to cancer. His theory is that when we eat or drink sugar, it causes insulin to spike, which may help fuel the growth of certain cancers, including breast and colon cancer. Dr. Cantley is so convinced of the connection that he has practically eliminated sugar from his diet. "I can remember when I was a kid the thought of eating bars and bars of candy was just absolutely fantastic. And now, if somebody offers me something sweet, I might take a bite of it to be polite but I would never finish it.

"I think the problem is a lot of people get addicted to sugar," he adds. Indeed, he thinks the dependency may be strong enough that people need to move slowly to break the hold. "If you take sugar out of your diet, maybe it has to be done gradually."

So we've got a weight problem in this country, and the same foods that are making us fat are also causing serious diseases. What are the solutions? I think it's safe to say that some combination of personal responsibility, education, and changing the food environment in this country offers our best hope. "At the end of the day, what each of us does with our feet and our forks is up to us, and so we do have to share in the responsibility for the solution," said David Katz. "Most of us who manage to be thin are working really hard to make it so, and have a skill set that the rest of the world doesn't have."

I totally agree with that. I've found an incredible amount of inspiration, smart advice, and new skills from the friends, colleagues, nutritionists, scientists, and other experts dealing with food issues whom Diane and I spoke with as we were writing this book. But making the commitment to get to a healthy thin is a lot harder if we don't know what's in our food. So one very important public health step is to require more informative food labels in both supermarket and restaurant foods, including a clear indication of how much sugar is added.

As an illustration, Stanhope points to the label on a yogurt container. "I think the time has come for the companies to have to say 'added sugar' versus 'total sugar' on the container, so we can differentiate between the sugar that is in the fruit or the milk, and the sugar that is added in the processing," she says.

That's just one example of the big-picture solutions Diane and I discuss later in this book. We can't hope to get on the right track as individuals until we get on the right track as a nation. We need smarter policies and healthier communities if we are going to really solve our problems with food and weight.

CHAPTER FIVE

FIGHTING THE FOOD DEMONS

My story, with Joe Scarborough,
Dr. Nancy Snyderman, Frank Bruni

With Americans living in a food carnival and eating foods that may have addictive properties, it shouldn't be a surprise that so many of us have eating disorders. Many of these disorders lead to obesity, while others help us keep our weight down, but not in a healthy way, as I know all too well.

When I set out to write this book, I thought I was writing about problems that were in the past. In recent years, I have managed to maintain my tight grip of control most of the time. But now, at Diane's insistence, I am trying to release a little bit of that control and settle at a slightly higher weight. My goal is to develop a more relaxed attitude toward food so that I do not have to live at two extremes: feeling hungry most of the time and bingeing occasionally. It's hard, and the truth is that acknowledging my struggles with food has uncovered some bad influences and feelings that leave me on the edge of reverting to old, unhealthy behaviors.

—*mm*—

Joe Scarborough tells another story about me, and it's one that I hate, because it's so embarrassing. But I'm in "tell-all mode" here, so I won't hide it. This one happened when we were traveling. We do that a lot, broadcasting the show from around the country. We tend to have especially long days when we are out of town. Generally it means getting up even earlier than usual, in another time zone, and staying up late to attend events and meet people.

Joe says, "We were at a luncheon for about five hundred people in California, and I took one bite of the meal and thought, that's not worth the calories. I looked over at Mika, and this skinny woman who I had assumed just didn't like food, had in thirty seconds devoured the entire plate—the chicken cordon bleu, the sauce, the fries, everything. She probably inhaled about thirty-five hundred to four thousand calories in thirty seconds."

Joe watched in amazement as I pressed my fingers onto the plate trying to get the last of the crumbs. Moments later, we were onstage in front of five hundred people! Later, he said to me, "I can't believe you ate that." I was horrified, too, but it really helped Joe understand why I work so hard to hold myself back. "It hit me that she was struggling every single day of her life to not do what I would do, which is eat when I was hungry. She *lived hungry* all the time. Every six months or so when she was just exhausted and her defenses were completely knocked down, she would, without thinking, just start eating like the rest of us, except even more ravenously."

It hit me that she was struggling every single day of her life . . . She *lived hungry* all the time.
—*Joe Scarborough*

―――

Another story still shocks both me and my husband. I had taken an Ambien one night to get to sleep. With my crazy schedule, I need to do that sometimes. The drug can increase the likelihood of sleepwalking, and that's what I did—down two flights of steep stairs from the bedroom and right into the kitchen. Jim told me what happened next. He thought I was coming down to get a snack because I couldn't sleep. I said hi to him, and then I went into the pantry and opened this big jar of Nutella.

Nutella is made from hazelnuts, skim milk, and cocoa, and it's meant to be spread on bread. I love, love, love it. Really, it's my favorite thing in the world. Never mind that a couple of tablespoons have as many calories, fat, and sugar as a Three Mus-keteers bar. Never mind that consumers have filed a class action suit against the manufacturer, saying they were misled into thinking Nutella was a healthy breakfast for their kids to spread on toast. I wasn't thinking about any of that when I reached into a drawer and grabbed a spoon. In the next moment, I began devouring it as if I was the hungriest person on earth.

Then I seemed to say "the hell with that," as I put down the spoon and reached into the jar with my hand, scooping out the Nutella again and again, then licking it off my fingers. Pretty soon, the stuff was all over my face. I dipped in one hand, then both, again and again. As the Nutella spread up my arm, I licked it off there, too. After I finished the entire contents of the jar I calmly went back upstairs to bed.

The next morning I woke up, took a shower, and went to work, with no memory of the Nutella raid. When I got home that evening and saw Jim, he was like "whoa" and I'm like "what?" And he says, "Nutella?" and when I looked totally confused he said, "Oh my, you must have been eating on Ambien." Then I kind of remembered. I thought I had just been dreaming about eating Nutella, but I had actually done this in the kitchen in front of Jim!

To me, Ambien is almost like a truth serum. It frees you of inhibitions, allowing you to give in to temptations you are usually able to resist. The Nutella night revealed the intensity of my ongoing eating issues.

—*mm*—

That kind of behavior is obviously unhealthy, and I pray that my daughters will not be as consumed by food as I have been. Throughout my school years and the early days of my career, I was aware that other people also had food issues. But frankly, I didn't talk to them about their issues, or about my own. It took me a long time to see my own eating disorder as part of a larger picture, one experienced by many other successful people. As I became more aware of that, I recognized how important it is for all of us to share stories about our own battles with food demons, so we can help one another replace shame with support.

Maybe because Diane and I decided to go public with our struggles, a lot of well-known people have been willing to talk very candidly to us about theirs. While we were researching this book, we were both amazed to learn how common many of those stories really are. Sometimes, they are linked to coping with a terribly traumatic event. Dr. Nancy Snyderman understands that as well as anyone.

Nancy weighed 135 pounds when she entered college, just as Diane did. It was a reasonable weight for women at their height, which was about five feet eight inches. Not skinny, but healthy. She told us what happened to her near the end of her freshman year at Indiana University. "My roommate was working late on a really hard calculus problem, and she was getting help from the residential advisor. I remember saying, 'I'm going to bed, but I'll leave the door unlocked.'

"An itinerant was hanging around the dorm. He slipped in the front door behind a student who wasn't paying attention when she came in. Then he went down the hall turning doorknobs. And mine was unlocked. He raped me, and the next thing you know, I'm wandering around campus in the wee hours of morning totally disoriented."

It was 1971, and rape was mostly hidden from view. The campus police took Nancy back to her dorm room, where she took a shower, got dressed, and went to class. "There was no counseling, no talking about it, no nothing, so I turned to food. Food was my savior. I suspect that if you talk to a lot of women who have some kind of traumatic event in their lives, you'll find they turned to food for comfort. I found great solace in it."

I suspect that if you talk to a lot of women who have some kind of traumatic event in their lives, you'll find they turned to food for comfort.

—*Dr. Nancy Snyderman*

It didn't take long for Nancy to put on fifty pounds, her way of trying to disappear from view. It took her a lot longer, almost twenty years, to lose the weight. "Learning to like me was the same path as learning to be healthy; it was the same path as rediscovering my self-esteem," she says. "Going off to fat camp didn't help; depriving me of food didn't help. All it did was make me put food under my bed. I would order salad when I was out in public, and I would sneak the potato chips afterwards.

"Every person who has a food issue figures out how to game the system. I don't care if you're anorexic, you're bulimic, you're a hoarder—it doesn't matter if that's what you want to do. But the only person you hurt when it comes to food is you."

―⁓⁓―

Frank Bruni, now an op-ed columnist for the *New York Times*, is another person who initially kept his history of eating disorders secret, later making them public in his memoir, *Born Round: The Secret History of a Full-Time Eater*. Before becoming a columnist, Frank was the newspaper's chief restaurant critic for five years. Being a "professional eater" was a curious job for a man who acknowledged to Diane and me that he was a "baby bulimic."

In a telephone interview (ironically, conducted while his refrigerator was being repaired), Frank talked about his earliest experiences with food. "It was really more about how huge my appetite was. I was about two years old, and my mother wouldn't give me a third hamburger. I got so upset that I threw up." Frank told that story for two reasons: to illustrate his belief that some people are hardwired to be big eaters and "because it is a kind of odd, quirky bit of foreshadowing, since when I was in college there was a period when I was an actual bulimic." Like Diane, Frank tried "pretty much every diet you can imagine, including juice fasts and eating nothing but fruit for days at a time."

He, too, tried the Atkins Diet time after time, but it rarely helped him lose any weight. "It was a chronic dieter's behavior, where you ignore evidence and keep engaging in 'magical thinking.' It would do nothing for me, because I think for that diet to really work, it's betting on you becoming so bored with the monochromatic eating regimen that you won't consume that many calories," Frank explained. The diet does not require calorie counting, allowing you to eat as much of the acceptable foods as you want. "I love meat and eggs, and ate so much of them that it didn't work for me."

Frank turned to bulimia in college in a desperate attempt to be thin without feeling deprived. "One of the things I found so seductive about bulimia was that I didn't have the same sense of panic or sacrifice at the beginning of every meal," he recalls. "I thought, if my willpower fails me, I have this safety valve of throwing up what I ate and the calories won't stick with me."

Frank's reliance on bulimia didn't last long, but his struggle for weight control certainly did. One of his hardest times came when he was covering George W. Bush's race to the White

House. He was surrounded by food on the campaign trail, and very little of it was nutritious. "Every single meal was some sort of buffet or a bunch of stuff being thrown at us on the campaign plane," he recalls. "Some days it was just a constant level of fairly abundant eating, and then some days it was stress-induced binge eating after a really, really grueling day. I would feel almost like a drug addict's desire for a blast of pleasure and a release. I would sit down in front of my hotel minibar and eat the peanuts, then the Oreos and then the Pringles. Before you knew it, I'd eaten every stupid snack in that minibar."

Frank tipped the scales at 275 pounds. In those days, he recalls, he would allow himself to overeat "because I would tell myself the lie that tomorrow I was going to go on a diet, or the next day I was going to fast. I would end up giving myself permission in the moment to overeat."

> **I would tell myself the lie that tomorrow I was going to go on a diet, or the next day I was going to fast. I would end up giving myself permission in the moment to overeat.—*Frank Bruni***

Eventually, Frank learned the secrets to good eating that helped him break the constant cycle of dieting and weight gain. He lost eighty pounds, in part by redefining appropriate portion sizes, and he has kept that weight off. Gaining control over his schedule was key for him, because it gave him time to cook healthier foods and to exercise rigorously.

When the *Times* offered him the job as restaurant critic, Frank thought long and hard before accepting it, concerned about the potential impact on his weight. Ultimately, he decided he would be able to eat with enough restraint when he was not working that he could stay "on the straight and narrow." Ironically, he actually gained some weight after his stint as critic ended.

Like me, Frank has not entirely conquered his food demons. "I still have a somewhat compulsive relationship with eating. I mean, the desire to overeat comes along with some frequency. I'm not a slave to it, as I once was, but I still have to struggle with it, and sometimes I lose the struggle."

—*m*—

The link between eating disorders and obesity is getting more attention from scientists. For a long time they were considered distinct. Conditions like bulimia and anorexia were viewed primarily as psychological issues, while overweight and obesity were viewed as either genetic or metabolic problems, or as failure to take personal responsibility. But now we are starting to understand that there is a lot of overlap, characterized by an all-consuming focus on weight and food.

This is where my story of food obsession and Diane's tale of fighting fat converge. Both of us spend an incredible amount of time focused on food. In Diane's case, she has lost weight, gained it back, and started all over again, virtually her entire life. In my case, I have been so terrified of that loss of control that I have resisted even weight gain that would be good for me. I would be healthier and more at peace if I weighed 135 pounds instead of 125, but I'm afraid that I won't stop there and the weight will keep on climbing. So I sacrifice and I suffer and I'm hungry a lot. What a waste of mental and physical energy for both of us. "At least your obsession with food helps you keep the weight off—mine doesn't," Diane told me with frustration. She may be right, but it is still not healthy. One problem is that being so thin really gets rewarded. When I'm at my thinnest, I have everyone in the world telling me how great I look. Companies send me clothes to wear, and I can't believe how attractive they are. I feel like a model. Women say to me, "You're amazing, look how good you look!"

That kind of praise drives me to keep my weight way down. It's hard not to enjoy so much reinforcement from the outside world. Culture is a very powerful force. Ever since I was a kid, I studied the landscape and I saw how things went for women—*prettier and thinner equals success*. Diane gets really annoyed when I say this. She thinks I am too willing to accept a culture where women are valued most for their looks. I agree with her that it shouldn't be that way, but it is, and that's a fact.

But I am finally realizing that trying to be extremely thin is like trying to collect water in a sieve. It just doesn't work. I have to come to terms with that. And when I hit the scales at 118, or even 125, that is just not healthy for me. I have more work to do if I am going to reach 135 pounds and still feel good about myself.

CHAPTER SIX

MIKA AND DIANE:
MAKING PROGRESS, STILL STRUGGLING

OUR STORY, WITH DR. MARGO MAINE,
LISA POWELL, SUE GEBO, D'MARIO SOWAH,
ANDY DEVITO, DR. THOMAS LANE

By the time we reached the halfway point in writing this book, Diane had lost forty pounds. Meanwhile, I was still driving myself crazy with thoughts of food and desperate to find enough piece of mind to achieve, and stop at, a ten-pound weight gain. I was still living hungry most of the time.

As I began confiding more about my eating habits and obsessions to Diane, she began pushing me harder to deal with my attitudes toward food and weight. She thought I was masking some of my emotional issues, instead of dealing with them directly. Finally, I agreed to talk with clinical psychologist Dr. Margo Maine, a nationally known specialist in eating disorders. Margo is also co-founder of the Maine & Weinstein Specialty Group in West Hartford, Connecticut.

Margo presented me with a completely different way of thinking about my eating patterns when she surprised me with a diagnosis of *orthorexia nervosa*. The doctor who originated the term, Steve Bratman, explained that "orthorexia nervosa indicates an unhealthy obsession with eating healthy food." The term derives from the Greek word *orthos*, which means "right," or "correct," and *orexia*, meaning "appetite," and is intended to sound like a relative of anorexia nervosa.

I was pissed off at first. Now I'm in trouble for eating too well??? As you can imagine, my first session with Margo was a little rocky. I have almost entirely quit the junk food that used to captivate me. And that's bad?

"We get so much information about food, and if you're health conscious it can kind of morph into an obsession," Margo explained patiently. "Lots of people get into that today."

Food, it seemed, was still owning me.

Orthorexia nervosa is part of a larger category referred to as "eating disorders not otherwise specified." Margo said, "In that diagnosis, people can have some anorexic diagnostic indicators, some bulimic indicators, sometimes they have a combination of the two, but they don't meet the full criteria for either one. Their concerns about their body and their eating are a driving force, so that's the unifying factor."

Margo said that some 40–60 percent of eating disorders fall into that nonspecific category and suggested my approach to food might put me there, too. "A lot of my patients eat really good foods," she told me. "They just don't eat enough of them, and they don't eat enough of the fats and other things that give you a feeling of fullness. When you get some fat in your gut the message goes back to your brain that you're starting to feel full, and it will help you slow down your eating." Without enough fat in my diet, I tend to feel hungry, so I have to use all this willpower to keep myself from devouring more food.

A lot of my patients eat really good foods. They just don't eat enough of them, and they don't eat enough of the fats and other things that give you a feeling of fullness.—*Margo Maine*

Margo said that most of her patients wake up thinking about food. Beginning first thing in the morning, they are already asking, *What am I not going to eat today?* or *How am I going to get rid of the calories I do eat? How much exercise can I get?* I can relate to that, because that's exactly what I do.

Margo thinks food has a lot of emotional meaning for me, and that my obsessive focus is far from healthy. She also thinks I am undereating given the demands of my very, very long day—a power job, two kids and a husband, lots of exercise, and an incredibly active lifestyle overall. She thinks I am not just hungry, I am starving myself.

At first it was hard for me to hear Margo talk about my relationship with food, because her approach is a bit too touchy-feely for me. She talked a lot about how I should love myself and let myself be happy, and that's not language I usually use. I'm also very uncomfortable assigning any responsibility for my eating issues to my parents because the truth is that they were wonderful and loving. I had everything most of us want to be able to give our kids: culture, travel, strong emotional ties.

Everybody in my family loved one another, and nobody screwed me up.

But it is true that I come from a dynamic, well-known family, and my brothers are successful and (I always thought) smarter than I am. That probably puts some pressure on me. "How we relate to food at this moment in time isn't just how we feel about food now; it's how we have used food our entire lives," Margo explained. "You talk about everyone else in your family being brilliant and your not feeling brilliant, about having some learning issues and feeling like you didn't fit in. Food was the thing that filled you up. You soothed yourself with food, and I think food still has that power for you."

How we relate to food at this moment in time isn't just how we feel about food now; it's how we have used food our entire lives.—*Margo Maine*

"I hope you feel brilliant now! I hope you feel successful now, because you certainly are both of those. But you may still be operating on that old relationship to food, which is 'I'm not good enough' and 'this will fill up the empty space.'"

I was resistant to some of her ideas, but in her patient way Margo helped peel back the layers of my psyche, and I began to get some important insights. One of her questions startled me, but I knew how to answer it.

"Have you felt like an imposter your entire life?" she asked.

"Definitely, totally," I blurted out. "I'm still an imposter."

"That's a common theme with a number of my patients," Margo responded. "They can be very accomplished, bright, and attractive. No one else would look at them critically, but they don't believe any of it is real." Her theory is that as women in this culture, we always have to prove ourselves, and part of proving ourselves is to have a perfect body and a perfect house and a perfect family. That rings true for me. I am always trying to please others. In my career I often did too much for too many people, just to please them and to be liked. It was a terrible cycle that was broken finally when I saw that I needed to recognize my real value, financially and otherwise.

Margo said something else that resonated with me. She said I seemed to be looking for balance and control in life, and wondered if controlling my food intake felt like a way to control the rest of my life, with its hectic schedule and huge number of commitments. Being able to eat well in a life with so much going on is really hard, and sometimes it seems to be the only thing I can really excel at.

"That's similar to a lot of women who, like you, are not in the throes of bulimia or anorexia," she said. "You are well enough and well nourished enough that you can live close to a normal life, but the amount of thought that goes into your relationship to food and the amount of planning and the degree to which your food intake and exercise define other feelings about yourself is significant."

It may be that my diet needs modifying, at least according to a couple of nutritionists we consulted. My typical daily diet consists of three or four meals, plus a steady supply of drinking water. I'm up by three-thirty in the morning and headed to work by four. En route, I'll eat one or two apples, and by six, I'll have a Starbucks Venti Misto, half espresso, half steamed skim milk.

My first real meal usually comes at about eight-thirty, and it's almost always oatmeal with flax seed, honey, and bananas. At lunch I'll generally have salad or soup. The large green salad comes with avocadoes and extra vegetables, but no dressing beyond a small amount of olive oil. If I choose a bowl of soup, it will usually be organic tomato soup or lentil.

Sometime in the afternoon, I'll have a snack, typically either Greek yogurt, a cucumber sushi roll, or a cantaloupe smoothie. For dinner, I often have brown rice and some combination of broccoli, spinach, Brussels sprouts, or cabbage. Other favorites include beans and brown rice, broccoli and tofu, or a sweet potato and a salad. I include a lot of tomatoes and avocado with some meals, and occasionally I will eat chicken. Once a week, I'll have a sautéed onion or spinach omelet, with five egg whites and one yolk. Usually I have whole-wheat bread with olive oil at dinner, along with a banana or apple.

I shared my typical diet with Canyon Ranch's Lisa Powell and with nutritionist Sue Gebo, who has a practice in Connecticut. Neither of them was very pleased. "Yikes—this seems pretty restrictive to me!" Lisa said. She estimated that I ate about 1,200 calories a day, not enough for someone who exercises and considers this a maintenance menu, not a weight-loss plan.

I shared my typical diet with Canyon Ranch's Lisa Powell . . . "Yikes—this seems pretty restrictive to me!" Lisa said.—*Mika*

Both nutritionists thought I should add more calories and more variety to my diet. They felt I was eating inadequate amounts of all three major nutrients—protein, fat, and carbohydrates—and said I'd feel better and have more energy if I increased my intake.

Lisa's biggest concern was that I was getting very little protein on most days. She encouraged me to include at least two ounces of lean animal protein, or some form of plant-based protein, with both lunch and dinner. Adding beans, a hardboiled egg, tofu, chicken, or fish to both my lunch salad and dinner meal would be an easy way to do this, she suggested. Lisa also encouraged me to include a little more fat in my meals, primarily extra olive oil, nuts, seeds, or avocado. She also wanted me to take a multivitamin-mineral supplement because she didn't think I could meet my most basic nutritional needs on so few calories.

Sue Gebo agreed, noting that "there are several missing items that would affect satiety." My afternoon snack did not have the right balance of protein and carbs, she said. The sushi roll had no protein, the yogurt had no starch, and the cantaloupe smoothie had neither one, unless I added milk or yogurt to it. Likewise, Sue said that my dinners needed a better balance of protein and carbs, along with some fat.

"It is no surprise that this meal pattern leaves Mika hungry," she told Diane. Her prescription was clear: I needed more food! "The omelet is a good idea, but with bread or some other starch. She would benefit from a more in-depth analysis of her intake (provided there are clearer portion sizes on her food record), a professional assessment of her calorie needs (which would require a detailed exercise record), and a meal plan designed around those needs to improve satiety and provide energy while preventing weight gain."

Lisa really nailed my problem when she encouraged me to include more variety in my food choices, and said I was stuck in a rut of "safe" foods. Adding new fruits and vegetables would not only ensure that I have a broader scope of nutrients in my diet, but also make my meals more interesting.

So it looks like my agenda is to adjust my diet and maintain my weight at a healthy level—not too thin, but not climbing steadily upward, either. Margo helped me recognize that if I can accept my "set point," my struggle will become a whole lot easier. Although my weight has been up and down since I was fifteen, I never fully realized that every time I gained weight I seemed to top out at 135 pounds. That is actually pretty reasonable for my height of five foot seven at the age of forty-five. Maybe that's the right weight for me now. It sounded so obvious when Margo and I discussed it. She almost has me convinced that if I just let myself reach my natural set point, I will not gain more weight.

Begrudgingly, I have to admit that our sessions have given me the freedom to nudge closer to that set point. I have let myself gain a little weight, and I am trying to feel okay about that. I'm trying to be less rigid about what I eat in the hope that I can get off the hamster wheel for good.

I am known for wearing body-hugging sleeveless dresses with very high heels on TV. I noticed the dresses getting a little too tight, and I was afraid the yellow one would pop open, live on television. I am now officially a size 4, pushing a 6, but stuffed into a size 2. Usually when this happens, I start running twice a day. Usually when this happens, I stop eating after 7:00 p.m. Usually when this happens I am very unhappy.

If you watch the videotape of the August 2012 Republican Convention in Tampa, Florida, and the Democratic Convention in Charlotte, North Carolina, a few weeks later, you will see something that has never happened in my twenty-five-year career. I'm not wearing my trademark sleeveless dresses as much (they were too damn tight). I'm in loose-fitting J.Crew button-down shirts and sweaters, comfortable Capri pants, and even more comfortable flats.

What you'll also see is a fuller face and even a little chin action. I hope you'll also see that I look happy—or at least comfortable with myself, and proud to be just the tiniest bit plump . . . in a good way. I have never been able to reach 135 pounds and feel this good before. In fact, I am shocking myself because I should be horrified at this moment. That's what I usually am when I hit 130 and a size 6. In the past, that's when I have turned and started the long road back to a size 2.

Believe me, I'm not completely at peace yet with what I hope will be the new me. I find that the tyranny of thin is never very far from reclaiming me. I still struggle with the tension between accepting a realistic set point and the need to please myself, my television station, and the public by looking picture-perfect.

I also have found that letting myself eat a little more "normally" has opened me up to fears that I will revert to past behaviors. Now that I allow myself a little more of the foods I like while I am on the road, the hunger pangs sometimes seem to grow worse. In fact, I am sometimes voracious. I am desperately afraid that will lead me to start bingeing again.

Obviously, I still have some work to do.

As I keep up my side of the bargain, Diane has managed to shave off sixty pounds with a weight-loss plan that seems solid. After signing up with D'Mario Sowah as her personal trainer, she is becoming much more physically active and following the healthy eating plan he recommends. She's on her way!

Here is Diane's account of what is going on with her.

The initial sessions at the gym were discouraging. I was so out of shape and so fat, I couldn't even get up off the floor mats without help from D'Mario. Fearful of losing my balance and falling, I felt like someone a lot older than I am.

But D'Mario was a rock of support. True to his philosophy at Akua Ba, he started from the inside out, working on my attitude first. "It wasn't the physical weight that I noticed when you started at the gym. I saw the emotional and mental weight," D'Mario told me later. Pulling me out of the emotional depths where I had landed was as important as helping me make progress physically, he said.

"I had to find words that were true and were encouraging to let yourself go as far as forgetting about the journey to lose weight, and just letting the process apply itself. That was the first thing I was thinking: let's get her to start. I didn't want you to be thinking, I've got to lose weight! I'm fat! I'm this and that and that! I wanted you to just think, okay, I'm going to Akua Ba, I'm going to take one day at a time."

With D'Mario's encouragement and Mika's cheerleading, it

started to work. I became a regular at Akua Ba, working out at least three times a week for at least an hour at a time. I was the fattest person in a room full of clients who mostly looked like finely toned athletes to me. But the workouts were so challenging I couldn't really focus on anything else. Using my considerable body weight as the resistance was more interesting and more difficult than using the machines I had been accustomed to at other gyms. Whether I was doing modified pushups and planks or pulling myself up from a nearly seated position, I was working hard.

D'Mario treated every bit of progress as though I had won the Boston marathon. The day I got up from the mat without his help he fell to the ground shouting, "She did it!" and beat his hands on the floor. Good thing we were the only ones there, but I was grinning like a fool.

He had such empathy and really understood the damage my weight had done, not only to my body, but to my mind. "What stuck in my head," he recalled, "was the story you told me about one of your speaking engagements where an audience member stood up and commented that you had gained a lot of weight. That always stayed with me. I'm always pushing my clients to be successful, but I feel a special dedication to you, because I never wanted you to feel like that again. Ever."

—⁓—

I was on the road toward weight loss again, but this time it had to be different. It just had to stick. Not only was I wearing plus-sized clothes, but for the first time I was really seeing the health damage my weight was causing. I started Mika's challenge in October 2011, and a month later my doctor put me on medication to lower my blood pressure. That was discouraging, but I clung to the hope that losing as little as 10 percent of my body weight could reverse that.

But there was something else; the nagging ache in my left hip, which had been diagnosed as bursitis, was becoming more and more painful. When I wasn't at the gym, I was nearly sedentary, nursing the hip with either heat packs or ice packs. It really hit me when my husband said, "Do you realize you haven't gotten out of that chair all weekend, except to eat and go to the bathroom?"

Honestly, I hadn't realized how much the pain in my hip had changed my life. I was turning down social and business invitations, because it took everything I had just to get through the day at work. I couldn't walk the dog more than a block or two. I'd been in pain for nearly three years and had tried physical therapy and medication. They had worked initially, but the relief didn't last. I was running out of options.

After my orthopedist took another X-ray, he asked bluntly, "Ever seen a German shepherd dragging its hind legs? That's hip dysplasia, and that's what you have. Eventually you will need that hip replaced." I was ashamed and embarrassed. Had my eating brought me to this point? Had my weight worn out my hip? The doctor never said so, but I was sure it was just one more shameful way I had allowed obesity to mar my life. At first I was afraid to tell my family, my friends, my colleagues, even Mika.

I got a second opinion, and when that surgeon told me the hip had been worn down to "bone on bone," I knew it was time. The soonest the doctor could schedule me for total hip replacement was February. I choked up when I told D'Mario about my impending surgery, sure that my plans to lose weight and meet Mika's challenge were crushed. I should have known that he wasn't going to let me drop out in despair. Instead he promised, "After that surgery, you're going to lose even more weight. You're just going to keep going, like a tiger let out of a cage."

D'Mario brought in a new trainer, Andy DeVito, who had experience in helping people recover from injuries and surgery. Andy spent several weeks prepping me for surgery, helping me strengthen the muscles around my hip and build strength in my upper body. It was another good match. Andy, too, was incredibly supportive and gracious. I asked him later about his impression of me, and he was very kind. "One of the first things I really noticed is your smile. Your energy was just so positive. I could see that you were working hard, and you were in a lot of pain, and I really appreciated the effort you were putting into this. I could see how hard it was for you to do the things most people take for granted, just being able to get up and down from the floor, get in and out of the car, or take a flight of stairs."

Andy is also a trained chef who specializes in healthy cooking, and he started coaching me on my eating. His dietary approach focused on reducing refined starches, processed foods, and alcohol. In their place he substituted lean protein, fiber, fruits, and vegetables, and kept telling me to drink a lot of water.

I was getting stronger, but my weight wasn't going down much, despite Andy's help. I knew that keeping a food journal could help keep me honest and aware, but frankly, I was too distracted to do it. I wanted to believe D'Mario and Andy when they told me the impending surgery would be a short detour in my progress, and that I would eventually get back on the road to wellness and weight loss. But in my heart I wasn't sure.

Just after Valentine's Day 2012, I got a shiny new titanium hip. Two hours after I was off the operating table, the nurses had me standing using a walker, and I took a few steps down the hall. At that moment, something just clicked in my head: I had been given a second chance, and I was going to make the most of it.

The next day I learned that eleven laps around the joint replacement unit were equivalent to walking a mile—and I set my mind on doing two miles. I did, with the whole staff cheering me on as I passed the nurses' desk again and again. I texted D'Mario and Andy with the good news.

"That brought a tear to my eye, I was so happy," said Andy. "When we're working with people, we take it very personally. And when a client does well, it makes me feel good about myself, too."

At the hospital, there was a daily afternoon reception for patients and their families. I noticed that several of the patients having hips replaced were younger than me, and some of them were very lean. They had worn out their joints through tennis, skiing, martial arts, and other sports. In talking to them I felt some of my shame melting away. Maybe this would work out after all.

I was out of the gym more than eight weeks, but Tom and I walked the halls of our condo building every day. At first I used a walker, then a cane, and eventually I was on my own. My friend Joan came and walked with me, giving me some security in those early days when I wasn't too steady on my feet. An occupational therapist showed me I could climb stairs again and so I did, several times a day. The pain was easing, and I was enjoying the walking. It still wasn't doing much for my weight, though. I had gone from 256 pounds at the beginning of my pact with Mika to about 248 by the time I was cleared by my surgeon to go back to the gym.

As I was healing from the hip replacement, I had to follow certain precautions, but Andy found plenty of ways to challenge me during our workouts. He created an integrated program with point-specific, body-weight rehabilitation exercises, such as hip abductions, which I could do while lying on a bench. We also worked on functional body movements incorporating resistance bands and medicine balls and other exercises to correct my body alignment.

For balance and lateral movement, we incorporated Pilates-based core and leg exercises and added boxing drills. We avoided getting down on the floor (a no-no in the early weeks of recovery) and instead focused on exercises I could do standing or lying on a bench. When we added elastic resistance bands around my ankles, I felt as though I had a sandbag weighing down my surgical hip whenever I did leg lifts. Andy promised that would get better, and it did. "I've always enjoyed puzzles, and when I look at the human body, it's just a puzzle to me," Andy said. "So my whole philosophy is looking at your body and saying, 'What can we do to take care of this? We needed to strengthen the surgical area, help you regain your balance, and work at reducing the limp.'"

Andy's faith that we could fix this, and that I would improve, made all the difference.

~~~

A few weeks into my recovery, I decided I needed another weight-loss plan. Akua Ba's healthy eating guidelines weren't dramatic enough for someone with so much weight to lose. The pounds were coming off too slowly. I needed a clean break: a way to change my bad habits, reduce portion sizes, and stop looking for that glass of wine every night. After all the diets I had tried and failed, I knew I needed more professional help and support.

I did some research and found a body of compelling studies that told me what I already suspected: very low-calorie diets do work, but they are best when combined with behavior modification. A behavior modification program most likely to lead to a permanent lifestyle change should include nutrition education, advice for changing patterns of eating, training in self-awareness and assertiveness, and instruction in coping techniques.

I turned to a program like that at the end of May. Offered as an alternative to bariatric surgery at the Hospital of Central Connecticut, the Take Off program limits food intake to 800 calories a day, taken in protein shakes, with a little fruit and some salad greens on the side. It's a drastic approach, but I had a drastic problem. The Take Off program generally lasts twelve weeks, but I am still on it after six months. It requires weekly weigh-ins, weekly visits with a nurse and a doctor, and a series of twelve hour-long classes on nutrition and behavior modification. Just as it takes a village to raise a child, it also seems to take a village, or at least a sizable team, to help me meet Mika's challenge.

As I listened to the other patients in the Take Off classes, I realized that our struggles are very much the same, although some people weighed a hundred pounds more than I do. They are men and women, some younger and some older than I am. Several are a lot sicker. A few are limping because of bad knees or hips, and a couple are toting oxygen tanks. I wondered how they had overcome the discrimination they must have faced, but it wasn't something we talked about. It's good to be in their company, because it reminds me of where I am headed if I don't lose the weight this time, and make it stick. I'll never forget the week when the lecture described the relationship between obesity and diabetes. "How many of you are diabetic?" the lecturer asked. Nearly every hand in the room went up, except mine. At least I had dodged that bullet.

The Take Off program has given me a chance to wipe the slate clean and to learn something new. And it's working. Who wants a glass of wine after drinking protein shakes all day? I'm not hungry and the salad greens at night are fulfilling my desire to sit down with Tom at the end of the day and share a meal. As the weight falls off, I am really encouraged and excited.

By the third week on the program, Take Off's physician, Dr. Thomas Lane, cut my blood pressure medication in half. The next week, my blood pressure readings were still good. I was starting to see another impact of losing weight. Week after week, the weight loss has been steady, though shockingly slow for a diet this restrictive. Two pounds a week at most, and for several weeks in a row only half a pound. But as I leave the weekly sessions, often heading to the gym, I try to concentrate on where I was when Mika challenged me, and how much better I am doing now. That's a lot more productive than dwelling on how much I still have to lose.

By mid-July, Dr. Lane had taken me off blood pressure medication entirely. Yeah!

—◦◦◦—

When I begin to move beyond the Take Off program, I will also need to learn how to eat again. Over the long haul, cutting back on processed foods and eating more plant-based whole foods is clearly the way to go. I will also need to relearn what appropriate portion sizes are, something I had really lost track of in the last few years.

By August, the other clients at the gym start noticing the change in me. One woman says, "You're glowing." She's right, and it's not the sweat. Andy has me boxing, and even though I am still a klutz, I am moving a lot better. Lateral movement, which was drastically inhibited by my hip pain, is so much better. I realize I am no longer afraid of falling. By mid-September I am down to 203 pounds. I've lost 40. I still have 35 more to go, and now Mika is upping the ante. She is redefining the challenge and telling me I should lose a total of 100 pounds! I might just do it.

Meanwhile, I have been reminded that weight is about a lot more than dress size and how I look. My weight was stealing my life from me, piece by piece. Refocusing on health, instead of size and looks, has helped me recognize that I have to make a commitment for the long haul. That's the only way.

Dieting does not work. I know, you've read that before, but it's really true. I should know, because that's what I've done all my life. I dieted my way up to weighing 256 pounds. No more. This time I am remaking my life.

CHAPTER SEVEN

IT'S HOW YOU THINK

MY STORY, WITH JOE SCARBOROUGH, DR. MARGO MAINE,
DR. DAVID KATZ, CHRIS LICHT, GINA BARRECA,
KATHLEEN TURNER, GAYLE KING, KATE WHITE,
JENNIFER HUDSON, SUSIE ESSMAN

To the outside world, Diane and I look as if we think entirely differently about food. I'm the one with the reputation as a thin, fit woman, the one always going on and on about the obesity epidemic; Diane's struggles are a lot more obvious than mine. But as our stories have revealed, we are in many ways the same. When Diane talks about visiting a twenty-four-hour supermarket after finishing the late-night shift at the news desk and buying cookies, M&Ms, chips, and ice cream to eat later that night, I'm nodding. I've done that, too.

I am still trying to find the discipline my mother valued so much. My body is healthier, but my head? Well, I am still working on that. At times I remain trapped in my thoughts of eating, and Diane does, too. Until we can spring that trap for good, there are going to be setbacks in our attempts to develop a wholesome relationship with food. That's why it is so important not just to follow the stringent rules of a diet, but to make more fundamental changes in how you live—to change how you think, to overhaul what you eat and how you eat it, and to become physically active. We'll talk about all that in the next few chapters.

—*mm*—

I am in awe of successful women who manage to be free of the tyranny of food. The ones who connect with everyone in a room, while I'm busy thinking about how I can connect with another platter of food. I go to parties and see successful women like Arianna Huffington or Sheryl Sandberg or the late Nora Ephron, and they look so comfortable with themselves, so in command of the room. Meanwhile, I'm wondering how I can get another appetizer brought over to me.

There I am, in conversation with Walter Isaacson or Colin Powell, but my mind is so focused on those appetizers that I barely hear what they're saying. Instead I find myself wondering, *Where is that waiter with the mini hot dogs?* My eyes are on Powell and I am nodding with fervent interest, but with my peripheral vision I'm looking for the waiter, and with my brain I'm wondering when he might show up. I keep on discussing the conflict in Syria as best I can, but by now I'm thinking that I might just walk back into the kitchen and get those damn mini hot dogs myself! Then my frustration turns to sadness, because I catch Arianna across the room. She also appears to be having a fascinating conversation, but I bet she is right there with her companion, not privately plotting a trip into the kitchen.

Whether it is the sensory pull of those mini hot dogs or full-blown addiction, my thoughts can be totally distracting. That's less likely to happen when I have had at least a modicum of sleep and am working a fairly predictable schedule. The pull is not as strong then, and I don't overeat. If I get enough rest, I usually have enough stamina to keep my eating under control. Believe me, it takes a lot of mental effort.

"Mika's told the story about how she was fired from CBS on her thirty-ninth birthday. She thought that was the end of her career," says Joe Scarborough. "She scratched and clawed her way back into the game, and then she decided she was going to take her health and her fitness and her body image to a whole new level. It was extraordinary watching her day in and day out sacrificing and suffering."

I'm not as able to maintain that sacrifice when exhaustion sets in, and that happens a lot in a day that begins with a 3:30 a.m. wakeup call. My demons come back to bite me, and I'm more likely to compensate for my rigid low-calorie diet by suddenly and swiftly scarfing down huge portions of food. Margo Maine says part of my problem is that when I'm exhausted I may actually need to eat more. My body is demanding more calories, she says, because "that's what our bodies need at those times. Our bodies go into these kind of emergency states, and we need to let that happen."

As I learn to accept that, it becomes easier for me to ease up a bit and eat a little bit more fat, a few more carbs, a little more of the fuel I need to keep myself going. In the past, my approach has been to resist and resist that call, and then to suddenly break down and grab every morsel in sight.

I am trying to think about the world more like Margo does.

"I believe that our bodies are gifts we have to take good care of," she says. "That means feeding them, not just restricting and being careful, but feeding and allowing them to enjoy life. Part of enjoying life is enjoying food to some extent."

—*mm*—

More than a year after our infamous conversation on Long Island Sound, Diane and I are more convinced than ever that sharing our stories and providing support to one another are huge steps toward changing the way we think about weight and food. They have certainly brought us closer to each other. "We need to be able to have that dialogue, but the first thing we need to do is lay down the burden of blame and shame," said obesity expert Dr. David Katz. "Until we do that, we as a nation are stuck at this impasse on obesity."

The first thing we need to do is lay down the burden of blame and shame.—*David Katz*

Katz knows it is not easy to be candid, but he insists it is crucial. "It's a good friend who will have that painful conversation with you, it really is. We need other people's support and their skill sets in helping us." That's why I've made such a point of talking about obesity during *Morning Joe*, although our executive producer Chris Licht was horrified when I first started doing it. "I was afraid it was going to turn people off because no one wants to get lectured about their weight by someone who's in such great shape," admits Chris. "But Mika has earned that right. She works hard to be in shape and wants people to be healthier."

Those of us who can reach an audience, whether on television, in the classroom, or simply at the dinner table, have an obligation to talk straight to people who will listen to us. We shouldn't be hiding from our own struggles, or denying the struggles of the people around us. Raising the issue of weight and insisting we deal with it together is an important contribution to changing our approach. That's why Gina Barreca, a professor of feminist theory at the University of Connecticut, starts her speeches by announcing her age and weight. "This way, the listeners don't have to sit there and try to do the math. Because we all know that women will look at a speaker wondering, 'Is she older or younger than I am?' and 'What's her dress size?' Until they can figure these things out to their satisfaction, they aren't entirely paying attention.

"I tell them I was born in 1957, that I weigh a hundred and fifty-three pounds. I explain that in an Armani I'm a size twelve, while at Dot's Dress Barn I'm a size twenty-two because, as women already know, the more you pay for your clothes, the smaller the size you'll be."

It makes sense to me. Women are always eyeing one another, so let's share what we're thinking about our own bodies and the bodies of people around us. That's what Diane and I are doing, and it's working.

—◆◆◆—

Some women seem able to take a much more relaxed attitude toward food than me, even if they have some weight they would like to lose. I especially like the way the amazing actress Kathleen Turner thinks. She knows as well as anyone about the demands on women to be thin, especially if they are in the public eye, yet she seems comfortable with a little extra weight on her frame. That can't be easy for someone who started her film career thirty years ago playing a siren in *Body Heat*. Some fans still expect her to look the same way. Her response: "Yeah, I know, I looked like that. I don't anymore. Okay? Get over it."

At the age of forty-eight, Kathleen played Mrs. Robinson on stage in *The Graduate*, and in one scene wore nothing but high heels. "For a whole twenty-two seconds," she added. "I think one critic said I looked like a football player. I'm like, 'I'm sorry? I mean, eight shows a week is not for sissies, guys.'"

After *The Graduate* had a successful run in London, Kathleen resisted taking the show to Broadway because she knew the nude scene would get a kind of attention she was not sure she wanted. As she was considering film options, she read a script that described the main character as "thirty-seven, but still attractive." She was so angered by that kind of narrow view of aging and women's bodies that she called the producers of *The Graduate* and said, "We're going to Broadway. I was forty-eight and it was, essentially, a real 'fuck you'—and I was very happy I did it."

Kathleen acknowledged that she is probably about thirty pounds overweight right now. Her gradual weight gain coincided with a diagnosis nearly twenty years ago of severe rheumatoid arthritis. "Before that, I was an extraordinary athlete. I did all my own stunts and absolutely loved it. The arthritis at one point put me in a wheelchair and the doctors told me I would never be out of it, at which point I told them that they were fired."

Numerous surgeries later, Kathleen has regained an incredible range of motion, and her younger co-stars on stage admire the physicality and energy she brings to every role. She thinks that at least some of the extra weight on her body has actually enhanced her career. "In some ways it's good for my work in the sense that I am, and always have been, a character actress. I'm fifty-eight and doing these wonderful, very strong, very eccentric women who don't need to please men anymore, right? In a way, the weight and the solidness of me enhances that."

When she's working, Kathleen is just not worrying about her body image. "On stage or on camera I don't think about how I look, because that could interfere, even block, my acting. I am fortunate in my work. I know that the pressure of weight and appearance is different to many women in their chosen work.

"I find it actually quite frightening to see some of the actresses on television now, because I don't know if they have any intestines. In order to look like that you have to spend every waking moment of every day thinking about your weight. That's a tyranny I don't want to accept. I really don't.

"Yes, I would be happy to lose ten pounds, and when I get off the road and back home, I will work on that. But I resent this demand that you have to look so incredibly, incredibly thin. It makes me angry. Who decides this?"

> **That's a tyranny I don't want to accept. . . . I resent this demand that you have to look so incredibly, incredibly thin. It makes me angry.**
> **—Kathleen Turner**

Gayle King is another woman who is able to accept herself and her body. She works hard to stay a size 10, and to keep her weight at 162 pounds. At five foot ten, she is the first to admit, "I'm no Skinny Minnie," but she doesn't get upset about it. She'll diet when she has to, and she'll exercise even though she doesn't like it, but she is just not fixated on weight.

Gayle radiates confidence when she walks onto the set of *CBS This Morning,* and her philosophy on food couldn't be more different from mine. "I've now gotten to the stage in my life that I deny myself nothing," she insists. "I'm not going to not eat bread, or not eat cake, or not eat sweets. I'm not going to live like that. So I eat exactly what I want, and if I fall off the wagon I know how to get myself back on the program, whatever that is."

That's amazing for someone like me to hear, especially when Gayle admits how much she enjoys food. She recalls some time ago being at a hotel and ordering a room service breakfast: scrambled eggs with cheese, bacon (extra crispy), and an order of pancakes. The menu indicated the breakfast came with toast, and when room service asked if she wanted potatoes, she said yes to that, too.

"I was giving the woman the order and she goes, 'For how many?' I was so thrown by the question because I'm thinking this is not a lot of food, that I said, 'Uh, two!'

"So the room service guy comes and brings it, and before he got there I had turned on the water in the shower and I said to the waiter, 'He's taking a shower, you can set it right here.' Then I called out, 'Honey, the food's here!' "

Gayle told this as a funny story, but to me it would just have been humiliating. She also told me about walking into the office of her news director when she was working at WFSB-TV in Hartford. "On the list of things to talk to me about I could see he had written 'Gayle's butt.'

"I remember thinking, damn, Gayle's butt? He says to me, 'On those wide shots if you could just push in, because your butt hangs over the chair.' I didn't even have the wherewithal to be offended. I'm like, 'Oh, okay, I'll watch that.' Now—and this comes with age—I know I could say, 'Wait a second. Wait a second.'"

In my own life, I truly love to run, but let's just say working out is not at the top of Gayle's list of favorite things to do. Actually, that's putting it mildly. "I hate exercise, I hate it, hate it, hate it, but I also know that it's necessary. People say, 'Don't you feel so much better after you work out?' Well, actually, no. I just feel that, okay, I did it. I did it, I did it."

I loved Gayle's stories because they told me so much about her. Yes, she does have to be aware of how much she eats, and she needs to push herself to exercise more, even if she doesn't want to. And, yes, there have been times in her life when her weight became a professional issue. She knows she can't ignore it, and she weighs herself once a week, using Jenny Craig, juice cleanses, or her latest discovery, Fresh Diet, a service that she says delivers really fresh, really delicious food to her home every day to shed a few pounds when she needs to.

But she's also okay with who she is, and how she looks. "I think my relationship with food is pretty healthy," she said. "It's a loving relationship, because I really think that eating food, sharing food, cooking food is one of the greatest examples of love."

I really think that eating food, sharing food, cooking food is one of the greatest examples of love.
—*Gayle King*

Because she is comfortable in her own skin, Gayle is also able to let go of the envy that sometimes accompanies insecurity. "There is always going to be somebody who's skinnier, who's richer, who's prettier. I discovered that years ago. Now I can see somebody who's gorgeous and I'm not envious. I'm like, 'Wow, I really admire what you do and who you are.'"

In the end, Kathleen Turner, Gayle King, and others remind me that what really matters is having a healthy mind and body. I'm all for a healthy thin, and I think women have to recognize that we are going to be judged, at least in part, on how we look, whether we like it or not. But some women are content to live with a few extra pounds instead of obsessing about what they eat all the time, and I admire them for it.

I also admire Kate White, who banned diet stories, normally a staple of women's magazines, while she was editor in chief of *Cosmopolitan*. "I just felt that girls have enough to worry about. Diets don't work. If someone promises you can lose ten pounds in four weeks you're going to lose it, but you're going to gain it back. I felt that it was unfair to women to keep fostering the notion of these quick diets, when really what you need to do is to overhaul your approach to food on more of a long-term basis. I decided if we gave any information about health and food, it would be just smart nutritional information."

Diets don't work. If someone promises you can lose ten pounds in four weeks you're going to lose it, but you're going to gain it back.—*Kate White*

The magazine does provide guidelines for eating smart, and under Kate's watch, *Cosmo* launched a new feature titled "Body Love," which is aimed at helping women feel good about their bodies. "That's a lot about celebrating your body and feeling good about it and feeling confident about it," she says.

Oscar-winning actress Jennifer Hudson is another woman who has been able to resist the cultural pressures most of us face. At any weight, she has always managed to maintain a healthy body image. "I remember the first time I was told that I was plus-size, at least in Hollywood terms. I was on the red carpet and the media were asking, 'How do you feel being a plus-size girl?' I looked over my shoulder like, 'Who are you talking to?' because I never saw myself that way."

Coming from Chicago, Jennifer thought of herself as just an average-sized woman. The norms of Los Angeles took her by surprise, but she didn't get thrown by them. "I was maybe a size twelve at the time, and that's pretty good. Where I come from, size is welcome. So I thought, hold on. I have the height of a supermodel, I have lips that people pay for, so why should I feel insecure? I didn't have those insecurities at all."

When she did decide to lose weight with the help of Weight Watchers, she was genuinely surprised by the attention it attracted. "I've had people coming up to me and saying, 'Oh, my God, you're my inspiration,' and I've thought, people were watching? I didn't realize that until after the fact." Curiously, Jennifer actually felt more pressure *after* she lost weight because her body began to get so much more attention.

Body image is also a nonissue for comedian Susie Essman. In my next life, I want to be just like her. Why? Because she tells it like it is, whether she's swearing a blue streak on *Curb Your Enthusiasm* or performing stand-up comedy. She's a woman who really knows her own strength. "As a female comedian, there's this tremendous balance of power and femininity that's very difficult to maintain," Susie explains. "It's a very masculine art form, it's a very aggressive art form, and it's very powerful being up there by yourself onstage. Stand-up is so hard, and I have to be so focused when I'm on stage that I don't have room in my head to think about what I look like while I'm performing." I can't imagine what it would be like to be able to worry only about what comes out of your mouth, not what your body looks like. It just doesn't work that way for most women on television or in show business. I take it for granted that I am always going to be judged partly on what I weigh and how I look.

"It would be a whole different thing if I was just an actress out there in the marketplace," Susie acknowledged. "But I'm a comedian. So it's different. I write everything that I say. I have my own sense of my own power because I'm onstage all the time doing that." Susie understood what it takes for me to get my job done, and I really appreciated that. "Let me tell you something, Mika. You sit up there with Joe and Donny and Bar-nicle, and you hold your own with them. You should feel pretty damn good about that. Because that's a boy's club over there, and it's not easy."

She also reminded me that it takes a lot more to succeed than a good-looking body, helpful though that is. "It's been said that a pretty face is a passport," she said, "but it's not. It's a visa, and it runs out fast. Yes, your life is easier when you're attractive; I absolutely believe that. I think things come more easily, whether it's standing in line at the deli or whatever. However, you'd better develop yourself, because there's always going to be somebody prettier, younger, and thinner. Always!"

> **You'd better develop yourself, because there's always going to be somebody prettier, younger, and thinner. Always!—*Susie Essman***

I know that, of course, but it's not always at the top of my mind when I am wondering how I look to the millions of viewers who are watching me every day. It's a way of thinking that needs to be part of our larger conversation, whether it is taking place in schools, libraries, or community centers, on television, or in political and public health circles. If we are going to get healthier as a nation, we need to think differently about body image, weight, and eating disorders. They are all so closely tied together.

CHAPTER EIGHT

IT'S WHAT YOU EAT,
AND HOW YOU EAT IT

My story, with Nora Ephron, Lisa Powell,
Dr. Cynthia Geyer, Dr. Nancy Snyderman, Kate White,
Dr. David Katz, David Kirchhoff, Christie Hefner,
Senator Claire McCaskill, Frank Bruni, Susie Essman,
Jennifer Hudson, Brian Stelter, Senator Kirsten
Gillibrand, Padma Lakshmi, Charles Barkley

As we were researching this book, Diane and I got an incredible amount of good advice about smart eating from our women friends (we found a few good men with tips, too). I really appreciated hearing fresh ideas about how to get over my obsession with food and weight. Diane, who has run through just about every diet out there, was also open to new ideas about healthy eating. Sharing strategies for losing weight, or maintaining a healthy thin, makes the journey a lot less lonely. True, at the end of the day, each of us makes our own decisions about what we put on our plates, but there's still plenty we can learn from others.

I especially appreciated people who were willing to be blunt with me, just as I had been with Diane. My late friend Nora Ephron was one of those. Never one to mince words, Nora

149

made it clear that she wasn't very happy with how either Diane or I approached food.

Joe and I had gotten to know the screenwriter, film director, and essayist quite well in the last few years. We'd been working on a project together: a romantic comedy, like others that Nora had already made so brilliantly. What we didn't know at the time was that Nora was sick. She was so optimistic about beating leukemia that she kept it from most people.

It is a tribute to Nora and her love of her friends that just weeks before her death she sat down with Diane and me to have a conversation for this book. She was as open and direct as ever. "I'll have what she's having," from Nora's film *When Harry Met Sally*, may be one of the funniest lines ever delivered in a movie, but in real life our conversation with Nora was not as hilarious.

Nora's fans and friends know what a foodie she was. When I went to Paris a couple of years ago, I got the full Nora treatment. She sent me a file of places to eat and told me what to order when I got there. "I love to eat," she told Diane and me. "I do nothing all day but think about what I am eating at my next two meals." I told Nora I think about food all day, too. But I don't do it with her joyful anticipation of wonderful food. Much more often, it is because I am trying desperately to stick with a tightly disciplined diet that often leaves me wanting more, much more, to eat.

"I've been up at night holding my stomach in hunger and crying, trying not to eat," I admitted to Nora. "And when I break down and give in to my cravings, it is not pretty."

"Boy, that's sad. That's so terrible," Nora replied. "Food is one of the great pleasures in my life."

Diane was candid, too, telling Nora how discouraged she had become in recent years about her inability to keep off weight after working so hard to lose it. Nora really drilled into Diane after she acknowledged dropping out of Weight Watchers. "Who told you you could stop?" Nora scolded. "You can't stop; it's like AA." Our conversation took place early in Diane's seventy-five-pound weight-loss challenge, and she got a little defensive, responding, "I never seem to be able to plan what I'm eating. I'm always grabbing something out of the refrigerator or on the run."

Nora would have none of it. "That's just an excuse," she countered. "You say, 'I'm always on the run and I can't plan my meals,' as if we are living in a place where we can't pick up the phone and get anything delivered to us in five minutes that's healthy." I cringed, knowing that Nora was right, but also that it was painful for Diane to hear. "I know how Diane is hurting right now because it is not that easy for her," I told Nora. "Having said that, she *has* to do this. This she and I have decided."

Nora agreed. "Well, we know it's not easy, but we also know that you can do it, Diane, if you just trust yourself to stay with it. Let's say you made a commitment that you would stay with it for a year. Right? I swear to God at the end of the year, you will have changed your eating habits."

—*mm*—

That's what we are both trying to do, and Canyon Ranch nutritionist Lisa Powell reminded us why it is so important. "The number one complaint in a doctor's office these days is lack of energy," she says. "I don't expect my car to run if it doesn't have the right fuel. How can I expect my body to have energy and to feel good without the right fuel?"

I don't expect my car to run if it doesn't have the right fuel. How can I expect my body to have energy and to feel good without the right fuel?
—Lisa Powell

Getting enough sleep is a part of fueling the body properly. Dr. Cynthia Geyer, medical director at Canyon Ranch in Lenox, Massachusetts, says that without adequate sleep, we become more stressed and that, in turn, makes good habits harder to sustain. "The very things that you might do to help yourself stay healthy kind of go out the window when you're stressed. You gravitate toward comfort foods; you forego your exercise, because you have to put the pedal to the metal and get your work done; you get sleep deprived." That becomes a vicious circle, Geyer said, and "you're hungrier, more stressed, and more resistant to insulin when you're sleep deprived."

Diane and I are persuaded that whole, fresh food is the fuel that powers us best. Staying away from supermarket and restaurant foods crammed with sugar, fat, and salt is rule number one. Unprocessed food is not always the easiest to get, especially if you eat out a lot, and it can take longer to prepare at home, but it's almost always the best. "There are no bad whole foods," declares NBC News medical editor Nancy Snyderman. "The bad foods are the ones that are manufactured and have words on the labels that you can't pronounce. You wouldn't purposefully eat arsenic. So why would you purposefully eat bad food?"

Beyond an emphasis on whole food, there is no one-size-fits-all diet that will work for everyone. Some people seem to do better increasing their protein and reducing their carbs, while others decide that a vegetarian or vegan diet is the best strategy for them. There are some tried-and-true techniques that help many people, but you'll have to pick and choose the ones that suit your own lifestyle and keep the cravings to a minimum.

For me, healthy eating is a matter of finding equilibrium. The diet that works best for my body seems to be a very careful balance of fat, protein, and carbs. The challenge I face is how to eat enough of the right foods so that I keep hunger at bay and maintain control without giving in to episodes of insane overeating. Kate White described her approach while at *Cosmopolitan*, which seems sensible to me. "I've really limited the amount of sugar in my diet, and I eat a certain amount of fat and protein. If you sit down to a dinner that involves chicken and cauliflower that has been roasted with some olive oil, and then something else, you're so satisfied that it's really hard to get a craving going."

What you should not do, of course, is latch on to every new food trend, or become a "serial dieter." Jumping from one diet to the next and the next and the next is "magical thinking," says Dr. David Katz. "There is no real magic, and people do actually know that," he told us. But "they turn off their common sense because their common sense tells them, 'The only way I'm going to lick this problem is to figure out how to eat well and be active, and since that's too hard I need an alternative.' They get involved in one boondoggle after another, with the Jiminy Cricket inside their head saying, you know this isn't going to work. But they drown that voice out."

Eventually, we have to start listening to that voice, because reaching and maintaining a healthy weight is a lifelong struggle. Anyone who has ever carried a lot of extra pounds probably has food issues that are likely to keep surfacing, at least from time to time. "This is not what people want to hear, but I strongly believe if you struggle with weight, you will always struggle with weight," said David Kirchhoff of Weight Watchers. "This isn't something you cure after twelve weeks."

I strongly believe if you struggle with weight, you will always struggle with weight. This isn't something you cure after twelve weeks.
                                        —*David Kirchhoff*

Kirchhoff has a term, *acting like a dieter,* for the short-term approach. "The weight comes off, you look better, you feel better, and you kind of get cocky. And you say, 'Awesome. I'm going to go back to my old life' and you regain the weight."

What we need instead is to make lasting changes. Christie Hefner, executive chairman of Canyon Ranch Enterprises, quotes from a line she hears often at the well-known health and wellness spa. "Canyon Ranch has an expression I love," she says. "Diet is a noun, not a verb." In other words, diet is a way of conducting ourselves over a lifetime, not an action to be taken at a given moment.

Missouri Senator Claire McCaskill eventually reached the same conclusion when she committed to losing fifty pounds. "Before, I was losing weight for an event, or I was losing weight for my wedding, or I was losing weight because I had just had a baby, or I was losing weight because I wanted to get into a pair of jeans," she admits. As Claire moved into her late fifties and required knee replacement surgery, her motives changed and she saw weight loss as a path toward "a full and fun and long life. I think it was age and feeling a sense of urgency about my health."

When it comes to deciding what to eat and how to eat it, personal preferences, culture and family, daily routine, and medical history all help define the approach that is best for each of us. Many people need structure to lose weight and keep it off: rules that tell them exactly what they can eat. David Kirchhoff calls it "going on autopilot."

"If you talk to anybody who has successfully lost weight and has kept it off, one of the things that they'll tell you is that, over time, they've learned to develop certain habits," he says. An example is "having the same healthy breakfast over and over again, so that it really doesn't become a decision anymore. You go on autopilot, and those habits allow you to fundamentally shift from an impulsive eating style to much more of a reliable, healthy eating lifestyle."

But the rules need to be of your own making, and they should make sense for your lifestyle. For example, Nancy Snyderman believes one of the biggest food myths is that you should not eat after 7:00 p.m. "It really doesn't matter, even though I know everyone thinks that's a no-no," she insists. Ultimately, the timing of your meals matters a lot less than what's in them. "Our bodies are a factory and you must run on a debit system. You've got to balance calories in and calories out. People metabolize things differently, diets are different, but at the end of the day, you have to know what you burned, and you've got to figure out what to put in the engine."

For Frank Bruni, learning to control portion size was the key. "I knew that where I'd always gone wrong around food was with kind of compulsive binge eating, and with taking a normal meal and upsizing it out the wazoo," he admits. When he became the Rome bureau chief for the *New York Times*, he conquered his big appetite by eating like a native.

"Italians eat portions that are much, much, much smaller than ours, and there's no similar embrace of junk food," he recalled. "Their pasta portions—in complete contradiction to the sort of American mythology of the big, big bowl of pasta with all these meatballs—are very, very restrained, and they just don't eat the volume of food we do."

Small portions, Frank said, "really do tug you into a more restrained place. This whole American fascination with getting more food for your money and that having its own intrinsic value? Italians don't share that. They really don't see that kind of gluttony as something to be embraced."

I asked Nora Ephron about her lifetime eating plan, since she had managed to celebrate the pleasures of food without becoming a slave to them. After gaining what she called "the freshman twenty-two" in college, she had an "aha" moment that set her on a new course. "I went over to see one of my fatter friends because I had a date, and I didn't have anything to wear, because none of my clothes fit me. I put on a pair of her pants and I couldn't zip them up. She started laughing at me in a way that just really pissed me off. I had her image in my head for the entire next year as I lost the weight and changed my eating habits forever."

How did she do that?

Long before the Atkins Diet had gained so much attention, Nora's forward-thinking doctor thought that high protein was the way to go. He said, "Protein, protein, protein. Protein burns fat." The same doctor also told her, "After you lose the weight, you have to diet for six more months so that you change your eating habits forever."

Another strategy in the Ephron household, and one that I applaud, is to dedicate your calories to food that tastes good. Nora said one difference she noticed between thin people and people with weight problems is that the folks who struggle with weight "don't know the difference between a piece of cake that is worth eating and a piece of cake that is *not* worth eating. We call this 'NWE' in our house—not worth eating."

Like Nora, Diane prefers a diet that emphasizes protein, and has in the past managed to lose a lot of weight on Atkins. Although its critics have been legion, a series of studies in recent years seems to vindicate that approach. The *Harvard Health Letter* called the diet "an antidote to the dumbed-down anti-fat message"[1] and recent studies[2] funded by the National Institutes of Health found that dieters burn more calories and maintain weight loss better with an Atkins-like program.

Susie Essman has taken a slightly different approach. "I've gone Paleo," she told me. The Paleo Diet, also known as the Caveman Diet, is built on a return to the days of our early ancestors. The idea is to give up most foods added since the agricultural revolution of ten thousand years ago, including dairy and grains. The diet is built instead on the traditions of hunter-gatherers and emphasizes fish, pasture-raised meat, vegetables, and fruits.

After thirty years of abstaining from meat, Susie's Paleo Diet has put meat back on her plate, and she says she feels "fantastic." Although Susie doesn't struggle with weight control, she does need to maintain her health and stamina to perform live onstage, and the Paleo approach works for her.

A protein-centered approach is not right for everyone. Christie Hefner is one of many people we talked to who believe the key to maintaining a healthy weight is simply fresh, healthy, and reasonably sized meals. "What we tend to do more than anything else is eat too-large portions and too much protein, as compared to vegetables, fruits, and grains," Christie says. "I haven't eaten red meat since 1974, although I don't believe that it's inherently unhealthy. I eat fish and chicken and a lot of fruit and vegetables and grains."

Christie's diet is built around unprocessed foods, eaten in moderation. "There really aren't any magic bullets," she emphasizes. "On the other hand, it's within all of our grasps to be pretty healthy if we are educated about what to do and are willing to make the effort."

Jennifer Hudson came to the same conclusion. She made a commitment to learning about nutrition after her son, David, was born. "My fiancé and I realized we didn't have that education as kids," Jennifer told us. "Food was always put before us and it was 'eat everything on your plate' and all of that. We didn't learn about a healthy lifestyle until we were in our mid-twenties. So we wanted to make sure we set an example for our son. And that's what really kick-started it for me."

Jennifer lost eighty pounds after signing on as a spokesperson for Weight Watchers, and is now the smallest she has ever been as an adult. "One thing Weight Watchers taught me: if you don't eat what you want, then that's when you tend to overeat. Before, I would think, I'm going to deprive myself of eating this, this, this, and this, but that only lasts for so long. Then you're going to go right back into it, and you're going to regain the weight, and you're back at square one. Now I can have cake, I can have pizza, I can have ice cream. But I know *how* to have it now. I used to order a stack of pancakes; now I have one."

Jennifer says she no longer feels that she is actually dieting. "I look at it now as my lifestyle. It feels like it's a part of me. You have to stick with it, and that's just the life choice that I decided to make."

Several people talked to us about getting someone to hold them accountable for their weight loss. Senator McCaskill is in the public eye anyway, so that made sense to her. "I've had a lot of cruel things said about me," she acknowledges. "You like to think you've heard it all and none of it bothers you, but there have been dozens of times that it's been very hurtful to read online comments where people say, 'She's got six chins,' or 'She might be vice president someday except she's too fat.'"

The senator took time from her heated 2012 reelection campaign to talk to us about the incident that changed her life. It was Mother's Day, and Claire was in her St. Louis home, helping her diabetic mother with her insulin injection. "One of my kids walked into the room and said, 'I better learn how to do this, Mom, because maybe someday I'll be taking care of you like this.'

"It was one of those moments that hits you like a ton of bricks," Claire recalled. "That this isn't about what size you wear. This is about physical health."

This isn't about what size you wear. This is about physical health.—*Senator Claire McCaskill*

Soon after, the senator embarked on a weight-loss journey that she shared with eighty thousand followers on Twitter. "I knew my weight and my appearance are part of the public domain anyway, so if I was looking for accountability, then it seemed to me it would make sense to turn to the public." One McCaskill tweet: I'M TIRED OF LOOKING AND FEELING FAT. MAYBE TALKING ABOUT IT PUBLICLY WILL KEEP ME ON TRACK AS I TRY TO BE MORE DISCIPLINED. OFF TO THE GYM.

I thought Claire was very courageous to put herself out there like that. She explained why she had. "I knew that if I went back to my old lifestyle, not only would I be accountable to myself for my own health, but I was going to be putting my public failure out there for everyone to judge." Besides, she got a lot of encouraging feedback from her tweets. "Thank goodness— for every hater out there, there are multiples of people who lifted me up and said, 'You go, girl' and 'You can do this.' So it turned out to be the right call."

Senator McCaskill called on weight-loss coach Charles D'Angelo to devise a simple eating plan for her. "I didn't do anything other than eat good food and use the treadmill five days a week," she says. Her mornings begin with a healthy fruit protein shake. Lunch is typically a Subway turkey sandwich or a salad with some kind of protein on it. At night she has a piece of fish or chicken with some green vegetables, and a fruit popsicle before bedtime. She snacks on raw almonds, and one night a week adds a few more carbs to her dinner meal "to give me a little boost."

The biggest change and the senator's best piece of advice: eat regularly throughout the day. "I was in the habit of thinking, oh, I've been good all day, I have eaten hardly anything. It's five o'clock, I'll go to this function and nobody will even notice if I'm having the raw vegetables with fifteen hundred calories of ranch dressing on them. Or I would decide, a pizza is okay because I haven't eaten all day."

I notice a big difference between Claire's first appearances on *Morning Joe* and how she acts now when she walks into the studio. In the early days, I thought she seemed tentative, almost defeated. "You know what I used to think about when I arrived?" Claire explained to me recently. "I was wondering which chair they're going to put me in, and then I'm thinking in my head where the camera angle is, because I want to make sure that my back shot won't reveal that roll of fat when I turn. Now I just think, oh, good, I get to come in and shoot the breeze with Joe and Mika!"

―――

Like Claire, *New York Times* reporter Brian Stelter turned to Twitter to support his weight loss efforts, sending a tweet every time he ate something. For a media reporter, it just came naturally to alert the world about what was going on. "On the days where

I ate what I should eat, I felt really good tweeting my diet. On the days where I made mistakes, I felt bad about it. That told me that the Twitter diet was working."

Sometimes it seemed like the "humiliation diet," Brian admitted. "On the days where I'd have two or three cookies, I was truly embarrassed to tweet it, and I would write that on my Twitter feed. I would say how embarrassed I was. But on the days where I was doing the right thing, which was basically just this fifteen-hundred-calorie-a-day diet, I couldn't wait to tweet it."

Nearly three thousand people followed his Twitter feed and encouraged him as he lost a hundred pounds. One California woman, whom Brian has never met, cheered him and scolded him—and lost fifty pounds of her own along the way. "People celebrated when I ate right and chastised me when I ate wrong. I needed to talk about what I was trying to do, and talk about my feelings about the food I was eating," he said. "It was helpful to talk about my suspicion that some of this food had an addictive quality to it, to make sure I wasn't the only one that felt that way. It's surprising how social the weight loss effort is for me."

> **People celebrated when I ate right and chastised me when I ate wrong. I needed to talk about what I was trying to do, and talk about my feelings about the food I was eating.—*Brian Stelter***

While Senator McCaskill and Brian Stelter put their struggles out to the public, Jennifer Hudson and New York Senator Kirsten Gillibrand kept them within the family. That proved to be another terrific way to get some support. When Jennifer started on her weight-loss journey, so did more than a hundred of her relatives. Together, they lost almost fourteen hundred pounds! One of her techniques was to write down everything she ate so that she was fully aware of what was going into her body.

Senator Gillibrand did much the same thing, keeping a food journal that she shared with her sister, who was also trying to shed pounds. The senator lost her baby weight, dropping from a size 16 to a size 6.

—*um*—

With my incredibly hectic schedule, I know as well as anyone how hard it can be to eat well at work and on the road. But Padma Lakshmi might have me beat in the challenge department, because as a host of *Top Chef,* she gains weight every single television season. Known as the first Indian American supermodel earlier in her career, Padma is also a cookbook author and an actress.

Diane caught up with her during a break in taping her reality TV show, which pits chefs against one another in culinary challenges. "I need to taste everything that these chefs have put their hearts and souls into in order to render a judgment that's fair," Padma says. "I have to eat whatever is put in front of me, so I put on about ten to fifteen pounds a season." It usually takes her about six to eight weeks to gain that weight. "I have a very talented wardrobe stylist who gives me clothes in two to three different sizes, so often I will go from a two to a six or a six to a ten."

While she is on the set, Padma says, "I don't think about calories. I enjoy the food. Then, when the show's finished, that's the time to concentrate on my health and the way I look. I don't try and do those at the same time, because it's impossible. You'll drive yourself crazy."

So what's her recipe for getting slim when it's over? "Make sure there's a balance in your life. If I've just spent six or eight weeks on the show, eating everything under the sun, the next six or eight weeks will be about really cutting back on fried foods, on cheese, on red meat, on alcohol, on starches, on processed foods. Eating healthy is like a bank account. If you spend your calories by eating a lot of them in one case, then you have to save your calories later by eating better. You know, it's just basic arithmetic."

Padma is one more voice touting the benefits of whole food. "Eating food as close to how nature made it is always a good idea. The more you process food, the less nutrients you get, the less natural inherent flavor you get from that food; to me, the less pleasure you get. If I eat a cucumber, I want to taste that beautiful green herbaceous flavor that smacks of the garden. If you eat processed food you don't really understand food, and I don't think you understand what you're putting into your body. And I want to know what I put into my body. My body has to last, you know?"

> **I want to know what I put into my body. My body has to last.—*Padma Lakshmi***

—*mm*—

Charles Barkley, the outstanding NBA power forward known as the "Round Mound of Rebound," offered us a story about the influence of culture on eating habits and how we can model change for others. Barkley always cut a bulky figure on the court, but at six foot six and 250 pounds, he played brilliantly. After he retired in 2000, Barkley gained about a hundred pounds. "I had gotten up to three hundred and fifty pounds, and my doctor said, 'There are three things that are going to happen. You're going to die, you're going to have a stroke, or you're going to have diabetes.'

"I said, 'I'm going to go out on a limb. None of those three are good.'"

His biggest mistake was continuing to eat during retirement as he had during his playing days. "I played in the NBA for sixteen years and I never worried about my weight. You're training for a few hours every day and you're playing games, so you can eat whatever you want." Weight Watchers came calling, asking Charles to be the spokesperson for its "Lose Like a Man" campaign. Charles agreed, but quickly came to his first hurdle: learning to eat fruits and vegetables. He had never eaten much of either one, unless he was ordering potatoes or corn.

Learning to eat pears or apples instead of potato chips was a major lifestyle change. But it's something he decided to do, not only for his own health but to serve as a role model for his home state of Alabama, which has the nation's fourth-highest obesity rate, and for the African American community. "We've got too many fat black people out there, plain and simple. We're trying to reach that demographic," says Charles. "Black people eat way too much fried food, first and foremost. I don't think we do enough exercise, to be honest with you. But the fried stuff is really the biggest problem."

The Charles Barkley Foundation hosts an annual gala in Alabama every year to raise money for health facilities for minority patients. "We started six or seven years ago, and we raised about twenty million dollars," he says. "We just opened up our first free clinic last year, actually, and my goal is to open up twenty of them around the state." The event organizer called him about the menu for the dinner they were planning for a thousand guests. "She complained, 'Even the vegetables are deep fried down here,' and I told her, 'Welcome to my world.'"

The dinner menu is starting to change, part of Charles' effort to approach overweight and obesity not just as an individual issue, but as a community issue. I really applaud his efforts, and I expect that he'll look great in the smaller tuxedo he'll be wearing at his foundation's next black tie fund-raiser.

~~~

Whether it is protein or Paleo, vegan or vegetarian, the emphasis on minimally processed whole foods seems to be a core component of maintaining a healthy weight. Structure and accountability are important, too, but you'll have to design a strategy that suits you: there is no single approach for everyone. Weight Watchers is "diet agnostic," says David Kirchhoff. "What we really provide is support to help people change their habits and their outlook," rather than advocating for one particular food or system over another.

What we really provide is support to help people change their habits and their outlook.
—*David Kirchhoff*

As usual, Nora Ephron offered the wisest bottom line:

It's one of the great passages to adulthood when you understand that if food means something to you, you have to watch what you eat every single day.

CHAPTER NINE

IT'S HOW YOU MOVE

MY STORY, WITH JOSHUA HOLLAND, CHRISTIE HEFNER, MAGGIE MURPHY, DAVID KIRCHHOFF

Changing how you move is every bit as important as changing how you eat. In fact, the two habits work closely together. According to the American Council on Exercise, if you diet without exercise, 25 percent of every pound you lose is lean body mass. When you lose lean muscle, your metabolism slows down, making weight loss even more difficult. On the other hand, the higher your percentage of lean body mass, the faster your metabolism—and the faster your metabolism, the more calories you can burn.[1]

I used to think of this as my antidote to bingeing. I would stuff myself with junk food and then exercise so compulsively that some people called me "an exercise bulimic." I'm not sure that's an official diagnosis, but it did seem like a good description of my manic ability to calculate exactly how far and how fast I would need to run to burn off a pizza or a pint of ice cream. I spent so much time obsessing over this in college that I barely managed to study, or even attend class. The same thing happened when I got into the work world. Early in my career, if I wasn't at the TV station working, it was a pretty safe bet that I was out running someplace.

I am no longer doing those internal calculations, and no longer spending all of my free time running. My attitude toward exercise is a lot less compulsive now, and a lot healthier. It's still a big part of my life, but in a very positive way. Honestly, exercising is how I keep my sanity and reduce my stress.

It's also how I maintain my health. Research tells us that regular exercise lowers the risk of early death, coronary heart disease, stroke, high blood pressure, type 2 diabetes, and even some types of cancer. Unfortunately, not enough people are paying attention to that message: the federal government's *Healthy People 2020* report estimates that nearly 80 percent of adults aren't doing enough aerobic or muscle-strengthening exercise.[2]

My strategy for fitting physical activity into my life is to make sure to keep moving, no matter where I am. Washington, DC, is the center of the political universe, so I'm there a lot for *Morning Joe*, and no matter how busy my day is I find a way to squeeze in some exercise. Every time I head to Georgetown for lunch, I go first to the *"Exorcist* steps," made famous by Father Karras' headfirst fall in the movie, and run them up and down. So far, at least, my head hasn't started spinning, and it hasn't caused projectile vomiting, but I have burned some extra calories.

I prefer to run outside whenever I can, rather than limit myself to the gym, and that allows me to exercise almost any-where. My friends, colleagues, and business associates know that I often return phone calls while I'm out running. I can get a lot done on that four-mile daily run, although I sometimes use it just as a "time out"—a chance to clear my head.

At home, I often add ten minutes of arm work with ten-pound weights to my routine, and three times a week I jump on the elliptical trainer for twenty-five minutes more. The whole regimen is pretty simple, and it's one that I can work into my hectic schedule, which is the key to doing it regularly.

My penchant for grabbing a little piece of my workout at every opportunity draws some chuckles among my crowd, but they have gotten used to it. They know that if we pass a steep hill when we take the show across the country, I might just whip off my heels and run up and down it a few times. It turns out that even celebrity trainer Joshua Holland, whose clients include Madonna, agrees that's a sound approach to staying fit. Although he is the director of training at the exclusive CORE club in New York City, Josh doesn't think exercise should begin and end at the gym. "Fitness includes everything from walk-ing to work to taking the stairs instead of the elevator," he says. His advice: "Move well and move often, and do as much of it as you can."

> **Fitness includes everything from walking to work to taking the stairs instead of the elevator. Move well and move often, and do as much of it as you can.**
> **—*Joshua Holland***

In a society where so many people work in sedentary jobs and power tools do most of our heavy work for us, we have to incorporate activity into our daily lives very consciously. I remember as a kid, we used to rake leaves for hours on fall weekends. It was just a routine, and we never thought of it as exercise. Now a leaf blower does the job in fifteen minutes with nearly no effort at all, and we don't get any health benefits. Maybe we should go back to raking leaves again. Or consider the trick that worked for Dr. Nancy Snyderman's daughter: she traded in her power lawnmower for a push mower and lost weight as a result.

—*uun*—

Nearly every weight-loss plan includes exercise, but just how much do we need? Federal guidelines recommend two and a half hours a week of moderate aerobic activity, combined with muscle-strengthening activities at least twice a week.[3] Healthy adults who follow those guidelines cut their risk of dying prematurely by nearly one-third. People who suffer from chronic diseases benefit even more, cutting their risk of premature death nearly in half. And the benefits aren't just for the body. Studies have shown that even moderate exercise is an effective antidote to depression, and a report by the Mayo Clinic indicates that it helps elderly adults ward off dementia.[4] But more isn't always better. My guiding principles used to be "the more I exercise, the more weight I will lose," but that's not necessarily so. A study from the University of Copenhagen compared three groups of men in their twenties and thirties. One group was sedentary, another worked out moderately for thirty minutes a day, and a third group exercised strenuously. At the end of thirteen weeks, the sedentary men weighed the same and the strenuous exercisers had peeled off about five pounds. But the "biggest losers" were the men on the moderate exercise plan, who shed an average of about seven pounds apiece.[5]

Food diaries showed that the men who exercised the most seemed to have gotten hungrier and ate more as a result. They also moved less over the course of the rest of the day. Those who were putting in thirty minutes of moderate exercise daily, by contrast, continued to consume the same number of calories. Just as important, the formal exercise seemed to motivate them to make changes in their daily activities, like taking the stairs instead of the elevator, and they had enough leftover energy to actually do it.

For most of us, that's good news: you don't have to train as hard as a professional athlete to lose weight and be healthier. What you do have to do is make the commitment to develop what David Kirchhoff of Weight Watchers International calls the "exercise habit." "Habits can be forces of tremendous good or forces of horrific evil," David writes in his blog *Man Meets Scale.* "How many of us drink a glass of wine at a certain time of day because it's just what we do? How many of us feel the need to have a snack on our lap when we watch TV at night, even when we're not hungry? These forces are deeply rooted in our neural pathways. However, if habits can get us into trouble, they can also be the force that makes healthier life permanent."

Psychologists say it can take as little as two months to develop a new habit. What if only sixty days stand between you and a healthier life? "I finally turned into a six- or seven-day-a-week exercise person, and it is the greatest gift of my life," David told me. "It's annoying to hear people talk about how their exercise is a gift to them, but there's some perverse truth in it, no matter how miserable I might look in a spinning class. It really does take time to make all these little tiny shifts in your life that culminate in a healthier way of living."

Jesse Fox, an assistant professor of communications at Ohio State University, is using technology to give people a powerful incentive to exercise. Her avatars, or "virtual humans," show people what a healthier, more fit version of themselves can look like. When she was a graduate student working at the Virtual Human Interaction Lab at Stanford University, Dr. Fox found that these doppelgängers were effective at modifying the behavior of their human counterparts. As participants in her experiments exercised, they watched their avatars lose weight and get in shape. When they cut back on exercise, their virtual "you" gained weight back. The study found that subjects with avatars exercised forty minutes more over the next twenty-four hours, compared to the control group. The avatars also influenced the way people eat, Fox found.

There is other technology available that is somewhat less futuristic, but also very helpful. All sorts of new devices can track your activity levels and measure just how hard you are working. I visited a friend in her office recently, and I was really taken by how great she looks. I said so, and she reached into her sweater and pulled out something that looked like a thumb drive for a computer. It was actually her Fitbit, which is essentially a pedometer on steroids. A little over two inches tall, and barely more than a half-inch thick, the clip-shaped Fitbit weighs less than half an ounce and costs about $100. You can carry it with you everywhere to measure how far you walk, how many stairs you climb, and how many calories you burn during the course of a day. When you synch the monitor with your other electronic devices, you can also get workout advice and plans from trainers and athletes.

Tools like this are coming on the market every day. Nike has its own device, called the Nike+ FuelBand, to keep track of your activity. Like the Fitbit, the bracelet tracks every step you take and every calorie you burn. It also lets you set activity goals and shows your progress throughout the day. "Tools like Fitbit and FuelBand make people more aware, and if that's the goal, then it's doing its job," says Josh. "If I look at my Fitbit or my FuelBand and I see that my points or my steps are considerably lower than they should be, I may go for a small run just to get those points up. Once again, that goes back to what? Moving more."

Becoming fit helps you come a lot closer to looking and feeling like the person you want to be.

Just eating less won't do it. "Everybody talks weight loss, but what you really want is a change in body composition, meaning less fat and preferably more muscle," says nutritionist Lisa Powell, who believes it is a mistake to focus only on calories. "If you are a large, pear-shaped body and you diet and lose weight, you're going to be a small pear-shaped body. If you don't like your shape, you need to exercise if you want it to be fit and lean."

**If you don't like your shape, you need to exercise
if you want it to be fit and lean.—Lisa Powell**

Canyon Ranch's Christie Hefner nicely summarizes my goal for both myself and my girls. "Your appearance should reflect you as a healthy person. That means that you're physically active and that you eat well, which I think are good areas of concern for girls, boys, men, and women, versus insecurities having to do with 'I don't look like that model' or 'I weigh too much.'"

**Your appearance should reflect you as a healthy
person. That means that you're physically active
and that you eat well.—*Christie Hefner***

Christie does Pilates regularly, works out at the gym, and loves to play tennis, ride her bike, and ski. "I've always paid a lot of attention to wanting to feel and look healthy, so I have been active in sports all my life. I was raised to eat healthy, and it was something I focused on."

She believes that magazines and other media need to show more images of vigorous women. When she was head of *Playboy*, she presided over a gradual change in the look of the women who appeared on the magazine's pages. "For many of the early years, you would never have seen athletic women in the magazine," she recalls. "That changed, not just in the appearance of women who were modeling in the magazine but in the appearance of actual athletes like Gabrielle Reece, a volleyball player, or Katarina Witt, the skater. We featured women with strong physiques, and they were both powerful and sexy."

Those kinds of images help to shift attitudes about what we consider beautiful and encourage the next generation of girls to value exercise. For some older women who did not grow up playing sports, and never developed the habit of exercising, it's harder to get started.

Maggie Murphy of *Parade* magazine was in high school in 1972 when Congress passed Title IX to ensure that girls have the same opportunities to play sports as boys do. "Team sports were not part of my era. I became an entertainment journalist because I sat home and watched TV and then figured out how to make a living at it," she laughs. Maggie calls herself a robust, hip-py Irish woman and notes, "There was a real disconnect in the past for women about how to lose weight. Look at Betty Draper on *Mad Men*, starving herself, then breaking down and eating voraciously. I want to say, 'Betty go out for a walk. You might be able to eat a little more turkey on Thanksgiving if you went for a walk.'"

Luckily, Maggie eventually did discover the benefits of exercise, even if Betty has not. She started with an aerobics class in college and eventually graduated to running, where she pushed herself to run a ten-minute mile. When a knee injury undermined that effort, she discovered SoulCycle, an indoor cycling class that combines sweat and inspirational affirmations from the class leader. Well-known devotees include Chelsea Clinton and Lady Gaga. Maggie calls SoulCycle her perfect exercise, and says, "I spend forty-five minutes sweating like crazy and I am set for the day."

I spend forty-five minutes sweating like crazy and I am set for the day.—*Maggie Murphy*

—*mm*—

A lot of people perceive barriers to physical activity that aren't really there. Two reasons some adults say they don't exercise, according to *Healthy People 2020,* are the cost and the perception that it takes a lot of effort. Neither turns out to be true. What exercise does require is discipline, and that's where Olympic athletes have something to teach us. We can't expect to reach their fitness levels, but we can match a little bit of their determination.

After training some of these elite athletes at the London Olympics in 2012, Josh Holland became convinced that discipline was the foundation of their success. "What I took away from that experience was how disciplined these people are. To me, that is what it boils down to. They were blessed with certain talents and physical attributes, but I think they have a talent in discipline as well."

Beyond making a commitment to exercise, your approach is limited only by your imagination.

When Josh posted videos on Facebook featuring a unique exercise every day for a year, he proved that neither a gym nor any kind of special equipment is required to work out. One of his favorite pieces of exercise gear is a jump rope; it's inexpensive and simple to use, and it fits right into your purse or suitcase. Most of his videos were not shot in a gym. "They were either in my apartment, or maybe out in a park," he said. "We all have a chair in our home, we all have a bed, we all have a sofa. That's really all you need. I've done exercises on chairs, including pushups. You can pick up the chair, you can curl with it, and you can do squats. Or how about just standing up on your own two feet and doing jumping jacks, pushups, or sit-ups?"

More exercise pros are getting away from workouts that require elaborate machines and focusing on what they call *functional movements*. Diane's trainer Andy DeVito used that approach to help her recover from hip replacement surgery and improve her fitness. "The philosophy is based on getting your body to move and work in ways that it was meant to, like climbing, crawling, pushing heavy objects; things that humans were designed to do," Andy explains. "A lot of the workouts we do simulate those movements and functions of the human body. We've stopped doing these activities because we're sitting at a desk all day."

Sitting turns out to be dangerous not only to our weight-loss efforts, but to our health, so that's another powerful argument for moving. An Australian study, based on twelve hundred participants, found that after age twenty-five, every hour of television you watch reduces your life expectancy by nearly twenty-two minutes.[6] So if you watch six hours of TV a day, you'll take about five years off your life. That's actually worse than the impact of smoking cigarettes, according to the report. And it's not the TV that hurts you, it's the sitting.

Other studies have confirmed the correlation between sitting and premature death.[7] The science is new here, and we're still not sure exactly why sitting for long periods is so harmful. One theory is that surplus "fuel" builds up in the body when we don't use the large muscles in our legs, because processes needed to break down fats and sugars slow down or shut off, and blood sugar levels rise as a result. We know that the average person burns 60 more calories an hour when standing than sitting. We need to do more research to really understand what's going on, but I'm alarmed by the findings.

Personally, I can't stand still, so this actually isn't much of an issue for me, but if you spend most of your work day at your desk, think about a few ideas for mixing it up. Stand up while you're making phone calls, keep the trash can on the opposite side of the office, walk around during your coffee breaks. Small changes add up and can make a big difference, both to your weight and to your lifespan.

Getting Americans moving again begins with the decisions each of us makes as an individual. But it doesn't stop there. And that's the topic we'll discuss next.

CHAPTER TEN

LEADING THE CONVERSATION

My story, with Dr. Nancy Snyderman, Kate White, Dr. David Katz, Rebecca Puhl, Dr. Ezekiel Emanuel, Rear Admiral Jamie Barnett (retired), Mayor Mick Cornett, Dr. Robert Lustig, Donny Deutsch, Senator Claire McCaskill, Senator Kirsten Gillibrand, John Banzhaf, Chef Lorena Garcia

The conversation that Diane and I have been having, and the ideas that experts have shared here about how you think, eat, and move, mirror the conversations I think we need to have as a nation.

Overweight people are in the majority in this country. We need to fix that, but we can't do it unless we are prepared to have an open, honest, and caring discussion—not one that stereotypes, blames, or disdains overweight people. The problem belongs to all of us, and so does the responsibility to find solutions. We need to face this head-on.

Morning Joe is all about conversation. By talking with people on all sides of an issue, we often find a meeting place somewhere in the middle, someplace we can settle, agree, and move forward. I don't think we are there yet on obesity, but there is a lot of constructive and public talk going on around the country. Many concerned people are trying to find ways to get us on the right track. I hope that hearing about their attitudes and policies can help us change.

If you'll pardon the pun, what follows is some food for thought. As I said at the beginning of this book, you won't agree with me on everything, and you may not agree with some of these folks either, but let's consider what they have to say. Some of their prescriptions just might work.

—*mm*—

A good place to launch a broader conversation about the national obesity crisis is to talk about the ideas we have about a healthy body. That begins with an honest look in the mirror. Although Hollywood stars may seem to be wasting away, most of us are not. "As the population becomes fatter, study after study shows that instead of feeling bad about ourselves, we have entered a collective state of denial about how big we're actually getting," writes health writer and blogger Tara Parker-Pope. "While researchers admit that some denial may have to do with personal embarrassment, the consistency of the findings suggests that neural processing and psychology probably both play a role."[1]

NBC's Nancy Snyderman thinks we need to get the word *fat* back into our vocabulary, and I agree with her. I know that Diane was very hurt when I first told her she was fat, but she now uses the term herself, and it is helping her face her own situation. We should talk about being fat, not to be pejorative, but because we have to tell the truth. By trying to be politically correct and socially sensitive, we end up skirting the whole issue instead.

Clothing manufacturers also help us do that, by allowing women to brag about wearing a size 0 or a size 2, according to Kate White, former *Cosmo* editor and author of *I Shouldn't Be Telling You This: Success Secrets Every Gutsy Girl Should Know.* "There's been all this downsizing in clothes. I ordered a pair of pants from a catalogue. I put them on and I was swimming in them. And I realized, what used to be my size has now been increased; it's still the same size but they've really blown out the waistline."

David Katz says that the tendency to tell ourselves little white lies is normal human behavior. "We tend to think we're an inch taller than we are, and we tend to think we weigh a bit less than we do," he observed. "We tend to think we eat fewer calories and we all tend to think we exercise a bit more than we do." When each of us admits the truth about our own body weight, we begin to understand that we have a shared problem.

At the same time, a lot of us struggle to respond in a healthy way to all of the media images suggesting that women who are beautiful must be thin. The average woman in America weighs almost 163 pounds and wears a size 14. So when Ralph Lauren hires a gorgeous six-foot-two model who is a size 12 as the face of his "plus size" line of women's clothing, he sends a message to every woman about what the fashion industry thinks.

"We have billion-dollar diet industries, billion-dollar fashion industries that communicate the message that women must try to conform to very unrealistic ideals of physical attractiveness," complains Yale's Rebecca Puhl. "Thinness has come to symbolize core values in our culture."

We have billion-dollar diet industries, billion-dollar fashion industries that communicate the message that women must try to conform to very unrealistic ideals of physical attractiveness.

—*Rebecca Puhl*

What's happening is that as American women are getting heavier, models and actresses are getting skinnier. Kate White recounts looking at older photographs of Christie Brinkley and Cindy Crawford and realizing that those models "were not skinny, skinny girls. They were very healthy looking, very feminine, and lush almost. When actresses became more of a fashion influence in Hollywood, they got skinnier, too. You look at Jennifer Aniston compared to how she was when she first started in *Friends*; there's a big difference."

Kate says that when she was at *Cosmo*, "I encouraged our team to use models that aren't super skinny. I reject superskinny models. I think it's important for us in the media to show women who are natural looking, who are curvy, who are more like the Christie Brinkleys who have luscious, healthy bodies."

I reject super-skinny models. I think it's important for us in the media to show women who are natural looking, who are curvy . . . who have luscious, healthy bodies.—*Kate White*

For Kate, it was a matter of showcasing good health—she didn't want to highlight a super-skinny body, but she was not keen on showing more plus-size models in *Cosmo* either. "I feel that we've run amok in this country with nutrition and food. And the way you deal with it isn't to say, 'Okay, well, we'll start showing people who are putting themselves in health danger,' just as I wouldn't show people smoking."

———

So how do we start championing bodies that are a healthy thin? For one thing, let's act on the latest science and start early. Dr. Zeke Emanuel tells me we should get kids on the right path even before they are born.

"We might think of in utero effects," he explains. "We know that a woman can have a big impact on the size of her baby and the amount of fat on the baby. We may need to think about pregnant women and the diversity and the nutritional content of what they're eating. We do have some good evidence that once you create fat cells, you can't really get rid of them, and therefore later in life it gets very hard—not impossible—but very hard to lose weight."

> **We might think of in utero effects. We know that a woman can have a big impact on the size of her baby and the amount of fat on the baby.**
> **—Dr. Ezekiel Emanuel**

If the tendency to be overweight starts in the womb, so might the craving for certain foods. But people can change their desires, according to Yale Prevention Research Center's David Katz.

"Taste buds are very malleable little fellers," he says. "When they can't be with a food they love, they very quickly learn to love a food they're with. They like what they're used to."

Taste buds are very malleable little fellers. When they can't be with a food they love, they very quickly learn to love a food they're with.
—David Katz

So here's the really good news: *research shows that taste buds can be retrained to like better foods in as little as one or two weeks!*

"Imagine if all that stands between us and one of the more massive opportunities in the modern history of public health is a hill only two weeks high?" asks Katz hopefully. "How do we help the public understand that they need a week or two to get used to it, and then they'll spend the rest of their lives being perfectly satisfied with a food that's much better for them?"

It's probably not quite that simple, as my own experience with eating mostly healthy foods and occasionally going on a binge suggests. But educating people at every opportunity can certainly help. The messages about food, weight, and health should be coming from lots of different places so that we hear them over and over again.

People who have learned how to eat well, enjoy their food, and maintain a healthy weight can share some of their secrets with people who still struggle. Supermarkets can help by installing interactive screens and other technology so that people know what's in the food they are buying. Some of the nation's leading grocery stores are already doing this, and others can follow. One innovation to adopt is the NuVal System, created by David Katz and his team, which scores food from 1 to 100 based on how nutritious it is. NuVal scores are placed right next to the price tags on store shelves, making comparisons easy.

Doctors also need to take more responsibility to educate their patients. Unfortunately, many of them don't even know where to begin, since only 30 percent of US medical schools require a nutrition course. Most graduating medical students say their nutrition education was inadequate, which tells us we need to do a much better job incorporating it into the medical school curriculum.[2]

Talking to parents about their kid's weight makes many doctors particularly uncomfortable, either because they don't know how, or because they realize it's going to anger some parents. "I can't tell you the number of parents who hate the doctor for initiating the conversation, like it's the doctor's problem," Dr. Snyderman says. "But it's the doctor's responsibility to be a child's advocate and call it as you see it. That means getting a kid help."

If an obese child or adult has a checkup, it should be the first topic the doctor raises. Instead, we have fat people walking into the doctor's office all the time and it never even gets mentioned. How is that possible? You don't walk in there with cancer and not have a doctor mention it. They take your blood pressure, check your temperature, check everything else, and weigh you. Then they should sit down and have a talk and explain how you can lose some dangerous weight.

That's more likely to happen when the businesses that pay for health insurance start insisting on it. A lot of companies are already experimenting with payment plans that reward doctors for *preventing* illness, instead of paying them for every health service they provide. Some are negotiating insurance contracts that encourage medical practices to improve the way they treat complex chronic illnesses. I'd like to see doctors make more money if they successfully manage interrelated health problems, such as overweight, high blood pressure, and diabetes, as a single package. I'm also in favor of reimbursing employees for seeking out nutritional counseling, and providing discounts on insurance premiums when a worker reaches certain health targets.

All of these are great ways to get people committed to improving their own health, while reducing the cost to employers. Put the right incentives together, and we can create a win-win.

—*mm*—

Obviously schools, where our children get 40 to 50 percent of their daily calories, have a big role to play in educating the next generation about food, health, and weight, and in making smart choices available.

It may surprise you, but the military is taking a lead role in pushing for better food in the schools, and I applaud that. "When we have somebody show up at our doorstep who wants to get into the armed forces and they're overweight, we have to overcome eighteen years or more of lifestyle habits," says Rear Admiral Jamie Barnett (retired) of Mission: Readiness, the organization of retired military officers that promotes investments in youth. "It's pretty difficult. We really need to be able to start in early childhood with the right nutrition, the right fitness, and the right development in order to ensure that they have the best shot not only in the military but in the workforce in general."

> **When we have somebody show up at our doorstep who wants to get into the armed forces and they're overweight, we have to overcome eighteen years or more of lifestyle habits.**
> —*Rear Admiral Jamie Barnett (retired)*

It's not the first time military officers have stepped forward with their concerns for our young people. Barnett points out that after World War II, the military helped convince Congress to pass the National School Lunch Act. Back then, too many Americans were unable to serve in the military because they were underweight and malnourished. Now, too many young people can't serve because they are too fat, so the military is trying to get junk food out of the schools and exercise back in.

"This is a longitudinal problem with a longitudinal solution," Barnett says. "What we really need to do is start with the kids who are in preschool, kindergarten, and elementary school."

Retired top brass from all branches of the military are visiting schools across the country, and they tell me they are shocked by what they have seen. One school district in Kentucky didn't even have an oven in the cafeteria. "All they had were deep-fat fryers. Guess what they were fixing for their kids?" asks Barnett.

That's pretty basic. I could not have imagined a school district without a stove and other tools to make healthy food.

Along with equipping our schools properly, we also need to make sure that school nutritionists have proper training and authority. I'm not entirely sure what they are doing right now, but I think nutritionists should be holding seminars with students, cafeteria workers, teachers, principals, and school boards to talk about how to make the right food available.

I'm particularly enthusiastic about the kind of work that Venezuelan-born chef, restaurateur, author and television host Lorena Garcia is doing. Lorena goes into the schools to train the staff that actually prepares the food, encouraging them to be creative in making the small changes that can put a lot more nutrients into meals. "We're really giving them a reason, and motivating them to start cooking a little more with ingredients that they already have, just stepping away from processed foods," she says.

Everybody should have nutrition, weight, and health in mind when they make food-related decisions for their cafeterias. To me, allowing schools to sell soda, candy, and high-fat snacks in vending machines, or à la carte on the lunch line, defeats other efforts to serve healthier meals in schools. I'd like to see all of that prohibited.

And we have got to put exercise back into the curriculum. So many schools have cut way back on gym classes and recess, and some aren't offering them at all. "We take normally rambunctious children, send them to school, bolt them to chairs all day long so they can grow up to become adults we can't get off couches without crowbars, and we medicate them in the bargain," complains David Katz.

With all the emphasis on test scores, it's not always easy to sell schools on the need to make time for kids to exercise. But what if kids actually perform better when they have a chance to get some physical exercise during the school day? We should fund research to find out more about that. "Kids need to get up periodically and run around, period, end of story," says Katz, who is the father of five children.

Katz has developed a novel approach, called ABC for Fitness, which gets kids moving in class. "We developed a program where classroom teachers could dole out activity bursts right there in the classroom for three minutes at a time, five minutes at a time, eight minutes at a time, at their discretion, throughout the day, whenever the kids needed it," he explained. "We matched the activity bursts to grade level and subject matter, and pointed out to teachers how they could teach during the activity burst."

To see whether ABC for Fitness made a difference, researchers conducted a study of over a thousand schoolchildren, and sure enough, the ones offered activity bursts improved their fitness, were less disruptive in the classroom, and needed less medication for asthma and attention deficit disorder.[3] The program, which is free, is distributed in schools throughout the United States and can be used at home, too.

I love this idea. Kids need to move. They need to sweat. We should be insisting that our schools make that happen.

———

I'm also really interested in some of the ideas being discussed in urban-planning circles about designing communities for health. We should be thinking more about getting sidewalks throughout our towns and cities, providing safe parks that are easy to get to, and locating schools and businesses within an easy bike ride from residential neighborhoods.

Oklahoma City mayor Mick Cornett emphasized those kinds of strategies at the same time he put his entire city on a diet.

Cornett began his effort in 2005, truly the best of times and the worst of times for his city. Back then, Oklahoma City was getting some attention and respect, showing up on lists like "Best Places to Get a Job" and "Best Places to Start a Business." But that same year, *Men's Fitness* magazine published a list of America's fattest cities, and Oklahoma City was right near the top.

"It embarrassed me," recalls Cornett. He was even more embarrassed when he went to a health information website, typed in his height and weight, and discovered that he qualified as obese. "It took that website to point out that I was a part of the problem," he admits.

The mayor's first step toward solving it was to put himself on a diet. Then he persuaded a private donor to fund a health initiative, beginning with a website, thiscityisgoingonadiet.com, which offered everything from diet tips and shared journals to corporate challenges and exercise opportunities. Cornett called a news conference at the zoo, stood in front of the elephants and declared to residents, "We're going to lose a million pounds."

We're going to lose a million pounds.
—*Oklahoma City mayor Mick Cornett*

Forty-seven thousand people signed up, and five years later the city had reached its goal of one million pounds. It was a remarkable accomplishment. What made it work?

For starters, Cornett took a leading role in the conversation and talked about his own story first. If he was going to put his city on a diet, he knew he would have to be honest about himself in the process. "I had to become comfortable talking about weight loss, how personal it is, how sensitive it is, how difficult it is, and my own lifelong struggles to keep my weight off."

Once Cornett went public with his story, it was as if a light had been flicked on across Oklahoma City. Suddenly, obesity was "okay to talk about at the dinner table and okay to talk about over the backyard fence and at the water cooler at work and at church," he says. "Seemingly overnight, people were willing to talk about obesity for the very first time in this community."

The mayor did a lot more than talk. Cornett realized that like much of America, his city was ruled by the automobile. So he gathered city planners and asked them to reinvent the city; instead of catering to cars, he wanted to focus on people. As a result, he says, "We're putting brand-new gymnasiums in all forty-five of the inner-city grade schools; we're building health and wellness centers throughout the community for seniors; we're completing our bicycle trail master plan; we're putting in new sidewalks throughout the community; we're putting in a downtown streetcar system to get a head start on mass transit. We are designing a city that revolves around people and pedestrians."

The restaurant industry has embraced the cause, too. Chefs began offering low-fat options on their menus, and the fast-food industry now advertises its healthier meals and tells consumers how to make better choices.

Even with such a comprehensive approach, the mayor estimates it will take ten years to completely change the city's culture from one that fosters obesity to one that fosters health and wellness. But the payoff has already started. Oklahoma City is now on the *Men's Fitness* list of fittest cities in America, and the mayor says the changes in the environment have attracted an influx of highly educated twenty-somethings. Jobs have followed. A recent study named Oklahoma City the most entrepreneurial city in the country, with the most start-ups per capita, the lowest unemployment in the United States, and what Cornett calls "a boom economy."[4]

I totally agree with the advice Cornett offers other government leaders who want to emulate his success. "Most elected officials don't want to preach the message of what you eat and how much you eat because it seems invasive. Many government initiatives on obesity fail because they end up becoming just exercise programs. That shouldn't just be a message for overweight people; that ought to be a message for *everybody*. I think it's wrong to suggest that obese people can just exercise their way out of obesity. It's about what you eat and how much you eat, and we have not run from that message."

—◊◊◊—

New York City's Mayor Michael Bloomberg is another public figure who thinks that government has a really important role to play in turning back the tide of obesity. He's my hero because he has gotten out there, ignited a conversation, and has even been sued as he pushes to make this issue a priority.

Under his watch, New York City began requiring chain restaurants with more than fifteen locations to post the calorie counts of their food. At least twenty other cities have followed his example since the law went into effect in 2008. New York also banned trans fat, a solid fat that is a leading cause of heart disease. Other municipalities picked up on that idea, too, and after the ball got rolling McDonald's and some of the other fast-food chains decided to eliminate trans fat from all their outlets nationwide.

Bloomberg also called on the New York State legislature to impose a tax on soda. That failed to pass, but public health officials and researchers say it would have a meaningful effect on how much soda we drink, and I'd like to see other elected officials take up the issue.

The mayor's latest accomplishment was to ban sales of soda and other sugary drinks in containers larger than sixteen ounces in restaurants, movie theaters, sports stadiums, and other entertainment venues. The soft-drink industry, joined by other business groups, sued to halt that regulation in October 2012.

I really admire the example Mayor Bloomberg is setting because politicians just have to make this a priority. Some people accuse me of calling for a "Nanny State" by welcoming the government into our supermarkets and restaurants and now, with my support for the large-size soda ban, even movie theaters. But I contend that the government *already* plays a real big role in how we eat, especially through the massive subsidies it provides to big agriculture. So it is not a new idea to involve government, it's just a matter of changing the way we involve it.

"The fact is, we already have the nanny state, because we've already been told what to eat by the food industry," points out Dr. Robert Lustig, the pediatric endocrinologist who has called sugar a toxic ingredient. "If you ask me, we'd be better off with a nanny state that has public health, not private profit, as its motive."

We already have the nanny state, because we've already been told what to eat by the food industry . . . we'd be better off with a nanny state that has public health, not private profit, as its motive.

—*Robert Lustig*

―∿∿―

I think the federal government can do a lot more to join the conversation, and to demonstrate the leadership and political will to change some of the policies that promote obesity. We should all be pushing our elected officials to act.

Ed Rendell, the former Pennsylvania governor, and Donny Deutsch were on *Morning Joe* one day, and as we were chatting afterward, Donny said, "Can you imagine if we could eradicate obesity? Everything else would follow. Our health care costs would go down, and our health in general would be better. Everything would change in this country."

Can you imagine if we could eradicate obesity? . . . Our health care costs would go down, and our health in general would be better. Everything would change in this country.—*Donny Deutsch*

He's right, which is why obesity needs to be at the top of the agenda in Washington. I challenge our politicians to explain why it isn't. Someday soon, instead of saying "economy, economy, economy" we need to start saying "obesity, obesity, obesity." We've got to. Because, as Senator Claire McCaskill points out, the two issues are so closely tied together. "It would be a relatively painless way for our country to soar with a completely sound fiscal footing if we could put a dent in this increasing epidemic of us eating cheap food in portions that could strangle a horse," she says. "Making that food primary in our diets is going to break our country if we're not careful."

One thing our public officials can do is use the bully pulpit, just as First Lady Michelle Obama has with her "Let's Move" campaign, which is dedicated to ending childhood obesity. Her initiative includes commonsense strategies to educate parents, provide healthier food in schools, help children become more active, and make sure all families have access to healthy, affordable food.

I believe we also urgently need to change the nation's farm policy, especially the agricultural supports that make processed food much less expensive than most fresh foods. Robert Lustig maintains that our current approach to crop subsidies makes sweeteners so inexpensive that "80 percent of the food items that are available in the US food supply are currently laced with sugar."

With a lot of research indicating that sugar can make us sick, Lustig says the government winds up paying twice.

"The government paying for food subsidies is, number one, breaking the bank. We don't need these subsidies. We don't have the Dust Bowl. We don't have farmers who are in trouble. We don't have a hungry population that needs dried, storable food. Number two, all the disease that comes of it, the government ends up paying for in the form of Medicare and Medicaid. So no wonder Medicare is going broke."

Meanwhile, average Americans find it harder to afford a healthy diet of fresh fruits and vegetables, and schools struggle to find the funds to comply with new federal nutritional standards. That tells me we should think more about how government can help make good food less costly than bad food. As Dr. Zeke Emanuel says, "We're not going to be able to raise the cost of school lunches that much, given budget realities, and so we've got to think about how we can bring the price of the healthier food components down."

A lot of people tell me we can do that by overhauling the Farm Bill, which is the key federal legislation guiding agricultural policies in this country. Instead of rewarding huge megafarms, we should be giving more support to smaller farms, especially organic ones that supply local food networks with fruits and vegetables. If we want families to eat better food, that's where we should be spending public dollars.

I'm very encouraged to have Senator Kirsten Gillibrand sitting on the Agriculture Committee, the first representative from New York in forty years. She takes a vastly different approach toward food issues than senators who hail from states that produce commodity crops, especially corn, soybeans, and rice. I am with her all the way.

Gillibrand says she wants to "create a framework that's focused on having safety nets or insurance for farmers when they go through a storm or a bad weather condition that takes a toll on crops. What we're also hoping to do is enhance programs that are 'farm to fork,' getting whole foods directly into our public schools."

As a mom and a policy maker, Senator Gillibrand is also backing the federal Healthy Foods Financing Initiative. I think that initiative is one of the most important tools for nourishing the 25 million people in America who live in areas known as "food deserts"; that is, inner-city neighborhoods, rural areas, and other communities where good-quality markets don't exist and people don't have easy access to fresh, healthy foods. This legislation would provide grants to help existing grocery stores, farmers' markets, and food co-ops sell fruits and vegetables at affordable prices, and draw new food businesses into areas where they don't currently exist.

I also agree with the experts who say the government should require better labels on our food and more transparency in the industry so that people have a fuller understanding about what they are eating, and what it does to them. The US Food and Drug Administration is talking about revising the current label and requiring calorie counts to be posted more prominently. I also hope we will see more specific information about sugar content so we know just how much sugar is added to each serving of food. *New York Times* columnist Mark Bittman has another suggestion I like: put a traffic light logo on the label. A green light would be for food you can eat all the time, a cautionary yellow light would describe foods you should eat only once in a while, and a red light would warn about food that should be avoided altogether.

We also need to push our political leaders to get involved in refocusing the food industry. "We can't all go back to hunting or trapping or growing our own food," acknowledges Robert Lustig. Instead, "we need a new food system, one that works for the populace, one that doesn't overfeed them, one that doesn't cause significant chronic disease, and one that actually protects the environment. How is that going to happen when the only thing the food industry is interested in is making money?"

The answer is that government has to pressure food businesses, and for that to happen, Americans need to pressure their government. It's not a matter of what's in the government's best interest, it's what's in the best interest of the people.

I think that legal action against the food industry is one of the ways we can bring about broader changes. As more conversation about the causes of obesity and disease takes place, and Americans become more educated about the food system, this is beginning to happen. Some of the same lawyers who went after the tobacco industry decades ago are now going after Big Food.

"Fat and food have become the new tobacco," says John Banzhaf, one of the first attorneys to take legal action against smoking in the mid-1960s. Banzhaf is a public interest law professor at George Washington University and founder of Action on Smoking and Health. "Those legal actions against smoking had a lot to do with changing the mind of the public. In the fifties, sixties, seventies, eighties, even early nineties, most people blamed smoking solely on the smoker. It was his fault, it was his bad choice, it was his lack of responsibility."

Fat and food have become the new tobacco.
—*John Banzhaf*

To me, that sounds very much like the way we have looked at obesity.

Initially, nobody thought to lay blame for smoking on the tobacco industry. That began to shift, Banzhaf said, "as the revelations came out about how they promoted addiction, about how they lied, how they were underhanded. I think people began seeing that while personal responsibility plays a role, and people shouldn't smoke, at least part of the responsibility lay with those who were promoting it."

Again, I see a parallel with obesity and the aggressive marketing of fast foods. Still another similarity is that anti-smoking measures began to take hold when we discovered how adversely nonsmokers were affected by secondhand smoke. Likewise, as we recognize how the costs of too much weight affect us all, in higher taxes and inflated health insurance premiums, for example— we also recognize that everyone has a stake in dealing with the problem.

By mid-2012, twenty-five lawsuits had been filed against companies like ConAgra Foods, General Mills, and PepsiCo contending that they are mislabeling their products and thus misleading consumers.[5] These high-profile cases have forced companies to change, especially companies that value their public image.

"They are much more worried that this is going to hurt them than tobacco companies ever were," Banzhaf says. "Tobacco companies already wear a very, very black hat. The food companies are reacting to the fact that we are beginning to place a black hat on them."

While the tobacco industry couldn't make a less hazardous cigarette, the food industry has a wider range of possible responses. "When you sue the fast food companies they can do things. They *are* doing things," Banzhaf says. "They are lowering the calorie count in some of their foods. They have introduced more nutritious entrees. They have provided increased disclosure of fats."

Walmart is one of the leaders here, reducing the salt and fat in some of the food they sell. "They're the big gorilla, the single biggest grocery seller in the world," said Zeke Emanuel. "Their decision will first and foremost shape their private label, but after that it will also affect a lot of the other products they sell. And a lot of manufacturers are going to take the products that they're selling at Walmart and distribute them more widely. So I'm strongly anticipating a very big effect throughout the manufactured-food industry."

Still, I wouldn't expect the food industry to voluntarily make all the changes we need. The lawyers are still likely to have a role. And legal action will eventually lead to new statutes and regulations. "We will litigate until they legislate," says Banzhaf. "In our country there have been quite a number of movements, including the civil rights movement, which started with litigation, because there was very little public support for significant change. The only way to begin the change, to kick down the door, to arouse public attention, and then get legislative attention was through lawsuits."

Here it might be helpful to identify some of the new statutes and regulations which have already been sparked by the fat law suits. For example, New York City and then California required the disclosure of calories in foods at many chain restaurants, including fast food ones, and this requirement will apply nationwide in 2014 as a result of the Obamacare statute. More than two dozen jurisdictions now have a tax on or aimed at sugary soft drinks. Many states followed the example triggered by litigation in New York City and are restricting what foods can be sold and/or even brought into schools. Some jurisdictions are prohibiting establishing fast food outlets within x number of yards of schools. And, of course, New York City has banned trans fats in foods and limited the sale of sugary soft drinks in movies and many other venues to only sixteen ounces.

—*mm*—

I say it's time to declare war on obesity. I know it is not going to be easy to win, as Nancy Snyderman explains. "Never before has the human race been threatened by a profound overabundance of food," she says. "Cheap, affordable, toxic food that coincides with a loss of American sidewalks, the raping of public schools and taking away gym classes, and a technological environment that invites people to do more by doing less. It's the perfect storm of societal issues that I think will doom the next generation if we allow it."

> **Never before has the human race been threatened by a profound overabundance of food.**
> —*Nancy Snyderman*

We can't allow it. The problem threatens our health, our wealth, and our national security, and I'm convinced that together we can make the commitment to solve it. It will take education, government regulations, legal action, and commitment at every level of society, but tobacco showed us how much is possible. At one time, half of all American adults smoked; now fewer than 18 percent of them do. Turning that around took a combination of things.

"It wasn't just doctors talking to patients, it wasn't just getting rid of the advertising, it wasn't just raising the prices, and it wasn't just changing social attitudes and driving smokers off campuses," says Zeke Emanuel. It was all of that and more.

So it has to be with food, he says. "We have to get smaller plates, we have to get better labeling, we have to get the price differential reduced so that the healthy thing is not the more expensive thing. All of these things are going to be important in getting our arms around the obesity epidemic."

TEN WAYS TO CHANGE OUR APPROACH TO WEIGHT

- **Start talking honestly about what needs to change.** Hold constructive and public conversations about weight, body image, and how we produce, distribute, market, and eat food in America. Put the word *fat* back into our vocabulary and start using other blunt and forceful language. It's not enough to say "eat more fruits and vegetables." We also need to say "here are the foods that are killing us."
- **Publicize the costs of obesity.** The idea is not to stigmatize plus-size Americans, but to allow government officials and employers to break out their calculators and see whether programs to prevent or reverse obesity are worth the investment.
- **Insist that our leaders lead.** People with influence and authority at every level—in federal, state, and

local government, in the workplace, in the health care system, and in the schools—should help promote the broad changes that will get us on a healthier path.

- **Establish a federal obesity commission.** I'd like to see smart recommendations, based on science, coming from the top about how to build healthier communities, incorporate incentives for weight loss into our health care system, make healthier foods more affordable, promote behavior change, and much more.
- **Fund more scientific research.** Losing and regaining weight involves complicated biology, and we need to learn more about that. We also need to understand whether food really can become addictive and what messages will get people to act.
- **Overhaul the food climate in this country.** There are a million public policy opportunities to make a difference. For starters, we should change the crops we subsidize, eliminate food deserts, revise the food label, and levy taxes on soda and other unhealthy food.
- **Educate the public at every opportunity.** Our health care professionals should talk about weight with their patients, our markets should install touch screens to provide more information about what's in the food they sell, and people who have succeeded should share their secrets with those who have not.
- **Make our kids the first priority.** There is lots more we can do to improve the quality of school lunches,

teach kids more about food, and get them moving. Teachers should talk to parents about their kids' weight. And there is no excuse for selling sugary drinks and snacks in school vending machines.

- **Forge a healthful vision in small towns and big cities.** Let's make communities that work—with sidewalks, bike paths, easy-to-access and safe recreational activities, farmers' markets, and stores that have an incentive to sell fresh and healthy food.
- **Celebrate a healthy thin in the media.** Enough with the ultraskinny models. Let's show photographs of what real and healthy bodies look like.

CHAPTER ELEVEN

TEACH YOUR CHILDREN WELL

My story, with Dr. David Katz, Lisa Powell,
Dr. Emily Senay, Dr. David Ludwig,
Dr. Margo Maine, Dr. Nancy Snyderman,
Maggie Murphy, Senator Kirsten Gillibrand,
Chef Lorena Garcia

Let's go back into our homes now and talk about what else we have to do to get our children on the right path and keep them there. Nothing is more important to me, because I am passionate about preventing my daughters from struggling with food the way Diane and I have. It just takes up too much brain space, and it's too risky for their health.

I'll keep arguing for creating an environment that promotes a healthy thin for our kids. As I've said, schools, businesses, health care providers, and government can and should do a lot more.

But we can't hand off all the responsibility. We have to fight back together against a food industry that targets kids with billions of dollars in marketing, a media industry that tries to impose its own notions of healthy bodies on the rest of us, and a diet industry that says weight loss is easy if you just buy this or that product.

Teaching our children how to resist all that has to begin at home. That's where we can control the conversation.

We've got to take food back. We need to be in charge, to take ownership over what we buy and what we cook, and make it a priority, because it is going into our children's bodies and we have to make it healthy for them. As parents, we have an obligation to provide a firm grounding in smart eating so that when we send our kids into the world, they are as prepared as possible for the assault they will face. That's what it takes if they are not to become that generation of overweight and obese kids whose life span is shorter than that of their parents.

So how do we get our kids to eat well and to develop a healthy body image? What's the right way to talk about this with them? What do we say? What do we not say?

Talking about weight with your children is like threading your way through a minefield. Too much, and you worry that your child loses self-esteem or latches on to disordered eating. Too little, and you risk a child whose weight makes her a target of bullying and sets her up for a lifetime of health problems.

I turned again to the experts for their thoughts and guidance.

―――

Everyone agrees on two things: good eating habits matter, and parents need to model good behavior. "We use the term *junk food* as if it's an innocuous thing," says Dr. David Katz, "but it is the construction material for the body and the brain of that growing child of yours. We would not countenance building a house out of junk. We would not sanction driving a car built out of junk, and yet we look around every day at children being built out of junk and everybody's okay with it. There's something profoundly wrong with that."

> **We use the term *junk food* as if it's an innocuous thing, but it is the construction material for the body and the brain of that growing child of yours.**
> **—*David Katz***

Changing that begins with parents, says Canyon Ranch's Lisa Powell. Their role "is to choose and prepare a healthy menu, and to model healthy eating behavior that's neither restrictive nor overeating."

Lisa gets frustrated by parents who bring their children in to see her and say, essentially, "Fix my kid" without looking at their own eating patterns. "Sometimes I want to shake them and say, 'You brought this food into the house!' That's the mother and father's responsibility: to decide what is going to be available in the house and how meals are going to be structured."

Dr. Emily Senay agrees. "Take them to the store, shop in the vegetable aisle, let them help you prepare food, get them involved in the process. You can't stop them from eating junk food outside the home, but if you give them information and continue to model healthy eating behavior at home, eventually kids will eat more like their parents."

Take them to the store, shop in the vegetable aisle, let them help you prepare food, get them involved in the process.—*Dr. Emily Senay*

It has to be a family affair. I think Jim and I are doing a pretty good job exposing our girls to healthy eating. We are certainly trying to shape their attitudes toward food and expand the horizons of their taste buds by training them to enjoy fruits and vegetables.

The girls are more aware of good and bad food than I ever was. We discuss it a lot in our household, and they generally lead the discussion. I tend to hang back, because I don't want to add to the pressure already imposed on them from my job and my issues with body image. I'm sure they think that is just as well—teenage girls don't need to hear their mother tell them how to eat every second of the day!

But they do need guidance, and I am grateful that Jim takes an active part in these discussions and does a lot of our grocery shopping. He'll buy organic peanut butter for Amelia because she runs track, and we give the girls a steak once a week because they are still developing and need protein and iron. Jim and I don't eat red meat so we'll have a different meal, but that's part of the conversation, too. And we get tons of broccoli rabe and Brussels sprouts, which all of us share.

When I was their age, I was like a runaway beer truck around food. One of my issues growing up was that I wanted to eat American food, and I wonder if that made me feel like I was missing out on something. In my household now, we have an all-American diet, but it's a healthy one. And I don't think my children feel the kind of lack that I did.

I don't think they feel denied. Ours is not a "Food Nazi's" household, but we do shop carefully and we don't buy food that we don't want them to eat. We don't keep commercial cupcakes or sugary cereal around, but we do have granola without a lot of extra sugar, we have almonds, we have whole-wheat crackers. We even have windmill cookies, which have a certain amount of fat in them, but they're just not over the top. We don't buy potato chips and dip, but we do eat baked corn and whole-grain chips, and we enjoy salsa with them. We have all sorts of juices, but none of them are the processed sugar-filled ones in boxes. They don't have added sugar and they are organic.

One place we are strict is with soda. There is absolutely none of it in my house. None. As far as I'm concerned, if you wipe all soda off the face of the earth, this would be a better place. I don't see any reason why anyone should serve soda to their kids. It's like letting them drink candy. It's nothing more than liquid sugar, and as we've seen, sugar is poison.

Guess what I get out of that attitude? One kid who never drinks soda, and one who always orders it at the restaurant. I can live with that, for now. It shows that parents can't influence all of their kids' behavior (as if we didn't know that), but without soda in our home, I know they are drinking a lot less of it.

Two studies back up my strong feelings here. In a Boston study, 224 overweight or obese high school students were given either the sugary beverages they usually drank or sugar-free drinks, including bottled water.[1] That was the only difference between them; they got no nutritional advice, and they did not change their exercise habits. After a year, the kids in the sugar-free group weighed an average of four pounds less than the soda drinkers.

"I know of no other single food product whose elimination can produce this degree of weight change," said Dr. David Ludwig of Boston Children's Hospital and the Harvard School of Public Health, who led the study.

Similar results came in from a study in the Netherlands that involved more than 650 children, ages four through twelve. During their morning break at school, some kept drinking their usual sweet beverage and others were given sugar-free drinks instead. Eighteen months later, the children drinking the sugary drink weighed an average of two pounds more.[2]

—

Even with our crazy schedules, Jim and I try to have a sit-down family dinner with the girls at least a few times a week. It's not always easy to do, especially since I really want the meals to be home cooked as often as possible, but the research I've examined is too strong to ignore: eating dinner together is a good tool for helping kids avoid obesity and eating disorders.[3] Family dinners don't happen often enough in many homes, says Margo Maine. "Sometimes when a family comes into my office and I ask them about family mealtime, they say, 'We don't eat together' or 'The last time we ate together was the last holiday.'" That's especially troubling given the research that's out there to suggest that kids whose families ate dinner together three to four times a week may be more resilient against substance abuse.

"When you're not sitting down, parents aren't really feeding their kids. Everybody has to fend for themselves," says Margo. In that situation kids aren't likely to get a well-balanced meal, especially if they come home late after a game or another activity. "They're just going to eat something high in fat and sugar. That's what we're drawn to when we're really, really hungry."

Dr. Nancy Snyderman says it is not only a matter of *what* we eat, but *how* we eat it. "All of those subtle things about how we learn to eat—manners, conversation, portion control, cooking together—those things have been lost in our generation because we no longer sit down and have dinner," she says. "Even if you do drive through and pick up the food, please take it home and put it on a plate. You eat slower, you eat better, and you're more cognizant about what you put in your mouth."

Even if you do drive through and pick up the food, please take it home and put it on a plate. You eat slower, you eat better, and you're more cognizant about what you put in your mouth.

—*Nancy Snyderman*

But I want to see families cooking together again, instead of relying mostly on takeout and prepared foods. That's the only way to have personal quality control. Our kids ought to see us cook and help us cook, because we all learn so much when we buy food, handle food, and cook food together. That whole transaction has been lost for many families. Kids should learn how much oil goes into a recipe, and what good healthy ingredients are.

That's the idea behind Big Chef, Little Chef, a program created by chef Lorena Garcia. I'm a big fan because it gets parents and kids together to learn how to cook healthy foods and take back control over what they eat. "They end up loving being in the kitchen," says Lorena.

I know it saves time to let someone else do the cooking, and it's hard to make different choices with both parents working. But as Dr. Senay says, it can be done. "You've got to think carefully, you've got to plan, and you've got to continually push out the toxic stuff." I just don't think we should be passing on responsibility for what goes into our kids' bodies to someone else. To someone who doesn't care. To someone who will add tons of butter and fat and salt and sugar to a dish to make it taste good so that you'll buy it.

Maggie Murphy, who edits *Parade* magazine and *Dash,* a food magazine, agrees with us. She is on a campaign to get more kids and parents making meals together, and her magazines provide simple and healthy recipes to help. "I think there's some connection between childhood obesity and the fact that people have become very disconnected from cooking," she says. "My mother was too busy working to teach me to cook, and I think our generation has lost something. We'd have more family dinners if we could simplify cooking so we could fit it into our busy, busy lives."

If someone as busy as Senator Kirsten Gillibrand can do her own food shopping and find ways to interest her two young boys in nutrition, I don't think the rest of us have a good excuse not to do the same.

The senator talks a lot to them about what their bodies need to grow. "When I ask them what they want to drink, I always say, 'Well, milk helps you grow, would you like some milk?' Henry always says, 'Yes, Mommy, I'd like milk because it helps me grow.'"

The senator also gets four-year-old Henry to see how many colors he can put on his plate, giving him blueberries, red and green apples, and other colorful produce. "It really helps the kids understand that the more colors they have on their plate, the more vitamins and minerals they have on their plate."

Senator Gillibrand also invented a point system that has helped her older son, Theo, understand the quality of different food choices. "We'd rate foods from zero to ten based on their quality. So candy would be a zero, and chicken broth and broccoli would be a ten," she explains. "When he would ask me for foods that had very little nutritional value, I would often tell him, 'Well, you can have those potato chips, if you pick something that's a ten to eat before you eat the chips.'"

I think she's on the right track, because both her kids adore fruits and veggies.

Senator Gillibrand also looks for teaching moments. On Theo's birthday, she allowed the boys to choose whatever they wanted for breakfast. Theo had cereal and fruit, and then took a cookie on his way out. Four-year-old Henry decided to just have sugar for breakfast: cookies, cake, and candy.

En route to school, Henry fell asleep on her shoulder, and couldn't even walk into day care. "When he said, 'Mommy, I'm so tired!' I said, 'Well, what did you have for breakfast?'" That gave her a chance to explain that he needed protein, not sugar at breakfast, and that he would feel tired without it. Now, "when Henry asks for anything other than a healthy breakfast, I say, 'How did that sugar make you feel, Henry?' And he says, 'It made me feel tired.'"

Although I try hard to model a healthy attitude toward food, there is no hiding the truth about my own challenges from my kids, and I do worry about imposing an eating disorder on them.

I know that's a real risk. "We do see a lot of families with multigenerational eating disorders," says Margo. "That doesn't mean genes. It means the shared heritable environment. That would include how the family related to food, weight, body image, and appearance. How did they tolerate or encourage emotions? What did they teach about perfectionism? And was that child ever allowed to feel 'good enough'?"

Other risk factors for eating disorders are temperament, family history of depression, anxiety, addictions, and obsessive tendencies, according to Margo. Stressors, such as trauma, loss, or difficulty communicating, can also play a role. "It is the environmental influences that turn the tide; genetics are an indirect influence. In other words, nature needs nurture."

Margo had already suggested that I channeled the high expectations of my family and my own concerns about fitting in into managing my body. That's why I know it's really important to give my daughters the words to talk about food and body image. "When kids have ways of expressing those feelings, they are less likely to do that," Margo said.

I also need to be really careful about the messages that I send my girls, either consciously or unconsciously. "Mothers need to think about what they're projecting, even without saying anything about their kids' weight," warns Emily Senay. "Constantly dieting or any sort of disordered eating in front of your own children is not going to help them. It's going to hurt them. Women have to decide how they're going to be comfortable with themselves before they can really engage their children."

Lisa Powell agrees. "We live in a culture where thin is beautiful and mothers want their daughters and their sons to look a certain way. I think there's a real need for acceptance of a range of body types and styles," she says.

We live in a culture where thin is beautiful and mothers want their daughters and their sons to look a certain way. I think there's a real need for acceptance of a range of body types and styles.

—Lisa Powell

Parents also have to recognize that children have spurts in their height and weight, and we shouldn't get too stressed about them. "Girls have to gain weight in order to go into puberty," Margo reminded me. "Between the ages of ten and fourteen girls need to gain forty to fifty pounds and grow ten to twelve inches.

"That's a hard process these days when we're so attuned to weight and size. We're afraid that someone will gain weight as a preteen and be obese forever. We're making so many kids so horribly self-conscious about their bodies and fearful that if they eat anything at all it's against the rules, and they're going to get their parents' disapproval."

So how do I avoid that, but still keep my kids on track? Sometimes I am afraid that raising the topic of weight will promote an eating disorder, instead of helping them sidestep it. I know from talking with my friends that I'm not the only mom who feels that way. A lot of us worry about subconsciously sending negative messages to our daughters, or projecting our own fears onto them.

"But that's the same argument for not talking to your kids about sex. It's the misconception that if you talk to them they will then go out and be sexually active," said Nancy Snyderman. "Start talking in kindergarten. Don't wait until they're thirteen. This is all better if it becomes a part of your family conversations."

Chances are your children already know a child suffering from disordered eating. Emily Senay recommends being very direct and asking, "How does it make *you* feel when you hear that so-and-so is doing this? Do you feel pressure to do anything like that?"

If your child already has a weight problem, there's an art to talking about that, too. Focusing on health can be helpful, Emily says. "I think you have to opt for questions about health such as, 'Is this the healthiest way to be?' 'Is this the best way for you to run faster and hang out with other kids?'"

But before you even raise the issue, do some soul searching about what's going on in your home, and whether you need to make some changes there first. "What doesn't work is saying, 'Sweetie pie, you're fat, you've got to solve it,' but in the meantime the family's going on exactly the way they have," warns Nancy. "It's a little bit like your spouse has lung cancer but you're not going to quit smoking."

When you raise your concerns, remind your kids how much you love them. That was the approach Nancy took with her own daughter. "I want my heavy child to lose weight, and I've said to her outright, 'I need you to live longer than your mother. If you don't lose thirty pounds, I worry that I will outlive you. And you can't do that to me.' And she heard me.

"I said to her, 'You are an adult now. I need you to have a big, wonderful, fabulous life, and I'm worried that you won't.'

She listened, and she's made all these little changes in her life that have allowed her to drop fifteen pounds.

"I couldn't make it about being sexy; it couldn't be about comparing her to her sister. It had to be about the fact that I as her mother need her to be healthy because I love her that much. And she got the message."

The other part of the equation is making sure that exercise is a family activity. Yes, we've got to put gym back in the schools, too, but the commitment begins at home. We should start by making a vow to pull the kids away from the TV or the computer and do something active together every day.

That can be a challenge even for parents who are fit, because a lot of us confine our exercise to the gym. Not good enough, says Lisa Powell. "That just relegates activity to a finite period: I am going to be active now and then sit in front of the television the rest of the day. What kid doesn't want to go do something fun with their parents?"

I was raised in the tradition of Brzezinski family walks, and I admit they were sometimes hellish. My parents' idea of a good time was walking or hiking no matter what the weather, in rain, sleet, or snow. In fact, we once lost our dog in a snowdrift. I can remember walking and walking even when my feet were freezing. I can even remember getting a shot of vodka at age ten to help me warm up, after climbing straight up a mountain in bitter cold weather.

My parents considered that a great time. I wasn't so sure, but what I really remember is that we learned a lot about each other as we walked; there were some great revelations and conversations on those adventures. I thank them so much for making family activity and exercise an important value in my life.

Jim and I have done much the same thing with our girls since they were little. As a family, we take long walks, play tennis, and go kayaking when we can. The girls invented "Cajun Come," a game we play with our dog, Cajun, which gets the whole family running relays, laughing, and having fun together. Watch out, though; Jim and I love to run, but these days our teenager Emilie leaves us in the dust.

Saying the Right Thing to Your Child

Here are some tips from Margo Maine about controlling
the conversation at home.

If you say this . . .	Your child hears this . . .	Try this instead . . .
I'm worried about your weight.	Oh, now my mom thinks I'm fat and stupid, too.	How are things going at school? Are you stressed out or worried about anything? What could we do to make things better?
Don't eat that or you'll get fat.	I shouldn't be eating anything. I have to stop eating.	You know, every now and then we should look at what food choices we have in the house and be sure we have a range of choices, not just the easy junk foods to snack on. Do you want to help me with a grocery list?
You look fat in that.	I am an ugly, fat loser. Even my mom says so.	How are you feeling about your body these days? It's easy to feel self-conscious and pressured to look a certain way, but everyone has a different body type and different strengths. It's important to figure out how to enjoy your body no matter what it looks like—you are beautiful, and I love you "as is."
You can't leave the house in that.	I'm just never good enough—I should just disappear.	Just because something is in style doesn't mean it looks good on everyone.

		Do you want to shop to-gether to find things that help you to feel good about your body, or would you rather shop with someone else? Just know that I want to help you. I know these years can be awkward ones when it comes to how we look.
That's disgusting.	I'm disgusting.	I love how you handled . . . that conflict with a sibling/ helping your grandmother/ (anything other than a critical comment about eating, food, appearance, weight).
You're eating too much. Are you still hungry?	She thinks I'm a fat pig. I am so hungry but I'll stop eating if I have to.	Sometimes we eat out of habit, or anxiety, or stress. I know I do that. So it's important that you have people to talk to about problems. I will always try to listen, but if I'm not listening, try to let me know. Or you can always talk to . . . (safe people: dad, aunt, family friend . . .). And it helps to have a bunch of things to do when we are stressed, not just eating a favorite food. Let's think about how we can build some stress management techniques into this busy life of ours.

WHAT I'VE LEARNED TODAY

I am sitting in my home office, looking at a photo of my two daughters. Carlie, fourteen, is a freshman in high school. Emilie, seventeen, is a junior. Both of them have vibrant, wonderful lives, and they are so busy right now that they probably won't even read this book. But I hope they will read it eventually, and that it will help them understand me better, and know how deeply I love them. I wrote this at least as much for the girls as I did for Diane or me.

I've tried to be very honest here about how much of my time and energy has been wasted obsessing about food. I could have used those years a whole lot better by focusing instead on making a difference in the world. I would do just about anything to keep Carlie and Emilie away from the pitfalls of food obsession.

If you are a parent, you know that your kids see and understand much more than you give them credit for. I thought my struggle with food meant wrestling with my own private demons, but I found out it was a lot more visible than I realized. Carlie and I were in the doctor's office recently for her regular checkup, and we both weighed ourselves. "I weigh more than you!" she tossed at me, without seeming the least bit upset.

She got off the scale and popped back onto the examining table and added, "*You* have an eating disorder, so that's why you weigh less than me." She said it very matter-of-factly, with that cutting honesty that is something of a Brzezinski family trademark. I was about to retaliate with, "Do not be disrespectful to your mother," but I didn't. After writing this book, I couldn't argue with her. Not only was it still true, but I actually loved that she had the nerve and the insight to say it to me.

It dawned on me then that my daughter is healthier than I am. She is completely fine with her weight. Carlie looks good, she exercises, and she has a healthy appetite that includes plenty of good food. She enjoys eating, but she's not obsessed with it. Right now, her much greater passions are singing and horseback riding.

Emilie worries more about her diet, but that's because she's a runner and she wants to win all her races. She is concerned about eating foods that will provide the optimal nutrition for an athlete, not because she's worried about holding her stomach in.

I think that's fantastic. Margo Maine helped me think long and hard about the risk of laying *my* issues on the girls, and I have backed far away from pressuring them. They seem to be doing just fine, and that might be in spite of me, not because of me. They are going to be beautiful women.

━━✍━━

I want my girls to see me at peace with eating, and I might just be making progress in becoming a better role model. These days I'm eating more, and I don't feel hungry all the time.

Today I made myself a sandwich with three eggs, Swiss cheese, and arugula on two big pieces of wheat toast, grilled in olive oil. I didn't measure the olive oil and I didn't worry about the fat in the cheese. And I ate all three eggs, including the yolks.

Nora Ephron, it was just what you told me to do. I wish you were still here so I could thank you. I know you'd be happy that I am finally becoming less anxious about what I am going to eat next. Nora, you told me to learn to enjoy food as one of life's great pleasures, and I am trying to do that.

I want my girls to see me at peace with eating, and I might just be making progress in becoming a better role model. These days I'm eating more, and I don't feel hungry all the time.—*Mika*

Nutritionists Sue Gebo and Lisa Powell helped me a lot, too. Their comments about my very rigid diet, and their suggestions about how I can make different choices, helped widen my horizons. I am finding ways to make better choices, and I'm eating a greater variety of food, knowing that I can't starve myself and I shouldn't binge, either. I'm giving up the pain of trying to maintain an unnaturally thin body weight. I am wearing a bigger dress size now, and on my good days, I like it. On the good days, I feel a calm I haven't known before.

Anyone with an eating disorder knows how hard it can be to sustain good behavior. Trust me, I'm still obsessed with food, and I think I am still addicted in some unhealthy ways. But I can't let down my friends who were generous enough to share their wisdom with Diane and me, and I'm trying to follow their advice. Like Susie Essman, I am finding my power in my work, not my body image. Kate White and Christie Hefner helped me adjust my picture of what beautiful and healthy should look like. Gayle King reminded me that it's okay to live it up once in a while.

Like Susie Essman, I am finding my power in my work, not my body image. Kate White and Christie Hefner helped me adjust my picture of what beautiful and healthy should look like. Gayle King reminded me that it's okay to live it up once in a while.—*Mika*

I'm not sure my parents will be comfortable with some of what I've revealed about my ongoing struggle, but I hope they understand that the issues I've talked about here were of my own making. Mom and Dad are amazing parents, and did so much to expose me to the many ideas, options, and goals that a rich life can hold, including fantastic food. I always feel the urge to apologize to them for being such a difficult child, but maybe it's enough for them to know that Carlie and Emilie are getting back at me in spades. I suppose this is just the cycle of life shared between a parent and a child.

Diane and I are the products of an unhealthy generation. We began struggling with food early in our lives as the obesity crisis was emerging in America. The food industry accelerated its marketing, and no one of import stopped to consider the consequences. I didn't recognize how I had been trapped until Diane and I began this book. Talk about denial: I thought all this research and writing would help Diane get *her* life back on track. But she made me realize that I had a lot more work to do on myself in order to be able to help anyone else.

I finally took an unflinching look at myself and started a different kind of journey. I expect that I'll still fall back into unhealthy eating choices in the future, but I am more self-aware and less self-righteous when the topic turns to eating. I won't let my world be framed by food any longer. My obsession ends today.

Diane and I have come a lot further than we ever thought possible. Telling your friend she's overweight, and then paying for the tools she needs to lose weight, is at the very least a bit unconventional, and it can certainly threaten a relationship. But as Diane says, "That's vintage Mika."

As I've revealed in *Knowing Your Value* and *All Things at Once*, I rarely take the path most people follow, and things usually work out best for me that way, and sometimes for the people I care most about, too. Diane has lost 75 pounds, and she's seen a ripple effect in her life. Her husband, Tom, has trimmed down, too, and so have some of their friends. Even their dog has lost weight.

I am in awe of how Diane stepped *way* out of her comfort zone to write this book. I remember telling her that we would have to bare all to our readers, and I saw her eyes almost bug out of her head. Diane is used to putting a good face on everything she presents to the public, especially on *Positively Connecticut*, the show she has produced and hosted for more than twenty years. Neither one of us was sure her weight-loss journey was going to be such a positive experience.

But somehow, Diane made it into one. Owning up to the enormity of her issues with eating, and how they had damaged her life and her career, had to have been a gut-wrenching experience. I saw tears well up in her eyes during some of our interviews about weight and prejudice, and I heard comments that made me cringe, too. There were times when I thought she must hate me for putting her through all this.

But the risk was worth it, and we've bonded more intensely than ever. I urge everyone reading this to take the same kind of risk. Talk to your friends and the people you love—have the conversation about being obese. Confront them about their health and their weight, and then offer your support. Believe me, it wasn't easy for Diane and me, but it has been well worth it.

Talk to your friends and the people you love—have the conversation about being obese. Confront them about their health and their weight, and then offer your support.—*Mika*

I'm not going to shut up now. This book may be coming to a close, but our conversation together is just beginning. I'll continue to speak out about the obesity crisis in our country, but when you hear me talking about healthy eating on TV, know that I'm not the skinny know-it-all who knows nothing about food obsessions. Know that I am struggling, too.

As for Carlie and Emilie, they're beautiful just as they are. That's all they need to know. It took me way too long to understand that about myself, but thanks to my family and friends, better and more beautiful days lie ahead. With all my heart I wish the same for you.

NOTES

INTRODUCTION

1. Allison A. Hedley et al., "Prevalence of Overweight and Obesity Among US Children, Adolescents, and Adults, 1999–2002," *Journal of the American Medical Association*, June 2004. See also Centers for Disease Control and Prevention, http://www.cdc.gov/obesity/adult/defining.html.

2. "Too Fat to Fight" and "Still Too Fat to Fight," reports issued by Mission Readiness in 2010 and 2012, respectively.

CHAPTER TWO: THE VALUE OF A HEALTHY THIN

1. Alexandra W. Griffin, "Women and Weight-Based Employment Discrimination," *Cardozo Journal of Law & Gender*, Summer 2007.

2. John Cawley, "The Impact of Obesity on Wages," *Journal of Human Resources*, Spring 2004.

3. Shaun Dreisbach, "Weight Stereotyping: The Secret Way People Are Judging You Based on Your Body," *Glamour*, June 2012.

4. *Lots to Lose: How America's Health and Obesity Crisis Threatens Our Economic Future*, Bipartisan Policy Center's Nutrition and Physical Activity Initiative, June 2012.

5. James P. Moriarty, et. al., "The Effects of Incremental Costs of Smoking and Obesity on Health Care Costs among Adults: A Seven Year Longitudinal Study," *Journal of Occupational and Environmental Medicine*, March 2012.

6. Eric Finkelstein et al., "The Costs of Obesity in the Workplace," *Journal of Occupational and Environmental Medicine*, 2010.

7. *Understanding Childhood Obesity*, 2011 Statistical Sourcebook, American Heart Association.

8. Rebecca M. Puhl et al., "Weight Based Victimization: Bullying Experiences of Weight Loss Treatment-Seeking Youth," *Pediatrics*, January 2013.

9. Keynote address by Sam Kass, Centers for Disease Control and Prevention, Weight of the Nation Conference, May 7, 2012.

CHAPTER FOUR: FAT: WHOSE FAULT?

1. "Still Too Fat to Fight," Mission: Readiness, 2012.

2. Frank Bruni, ". . . And Love Handles for All," *New York Times,* April 16, 2012.

3. "Rudd Center Releases Unprecedented Report on Fast Food Nutrition and Marketing to Youth," *Rudd Center Health Digest*, November 2010.

4. Ibid.

5. David M Cutler, Edward L. Glaeser, and Jesse M, Shapiro, "Why Have Americans Become More Obese?" Harvard Institute of Economic Research Working Paper No. 1994, January 2003.

6. A. N. Gearhardt et al., "An Examination of the Food Addiction Construct in Obese Patients with Binge Eating Disorder," *International Journal of Eating Disorders* 45, 2012: 657–63; A. N. Gearhardt et al., "The Addiction Potential of Hyperpalatable Foods, *Current Drug Abuse Reviews* 4, 2011: 140–45.

CHAPTER EIGHT: IT'S WHAT YOU EAT, AND HOW YOU EAT IT

1. "Low Carb or Low Fat Diet? The Harvard Health Letter Investigates the Debate," *Harvard Health Publications*, July 2004.

2. "Study Compares Year-long Effectiveness of Four Weight-loss Plans," *Research Spotlight*, National Institutes of Health, March 2007.

CHAPTER NINE: IT'S HOW YOU MOVE

1. More "Fit Facts" about eating and workout plans can be found at http://www.acefitness.org/fitness-fact/13/Weight-Management/.

2. *Healthy People 2020*, US Dept of Health and Human Services, Office of Disease Prevention; Health Promotion, November 2010, download at www.healthypeople.gov.

3. "Physical Activity Guidelines for Americans," US Dept of Health and Human Services, download at www.health.gov.

4. Yonas Geda et al., "Aerobic Exercise May Reduce the Risk of Dementia," *Mayo Clinic Proceedings*, September 2011.

5. M. Rosenkilde et al., "Body Fat Loss and Compensatory Mechanisms in Response to Different Doses of Aerobic Exercise—A Randomized Controlled Trial in Overweight Sedentary Males," *American Journal of Physiology*, September 2012.

6. J. Lennert Veerman et al., "Television Viewing Time and Reduced Life Expectancy: A Life Table Analysis," *British Journal of Sports Medicine*, August 2011.

7. "Cutting Daily Sitting Time to Under 3 Hours Might Extend Life by 2 Years; Watching TV for Less Than 2 Hours a Day Might Add Extra 1.4 Years," Pennington BioMedical Research Center press release, July 10, 2012.

CHAPTER TEN: LEADING THE CONVERSATION

1. Tara Parker-Pope, "Are Most People in Denial about their Weight?," *New York Times*, April 18, 2012.

2. Mara Vitolins et al., "Medical Schools Fall Short on Teaching Students about Obesity," *Teaching and Learning in Medicine*, July 2012.

3. David L. Katz, "Putting Physical Activity Where It Fits in the School Day: Preliminary Results of the ABC (Activity Bursts in the Classroom) for Fitness Program," *Preventing Chronic Disease*, July 2010.

4. "Seven Most Business Friendly Cities," CNN Money, June 11, 2012.

5. "Ten Fat Law Suits (including 2 threatened ones) Have Been Successful—While One is Still Pending," http://banzhaf.net/suefat.html.

CHAPTER ELEVEN: TEACH YOUR CHILDREN WELL

1. Deborah Kotz, "Limits on sugary drinks backed by research," *Boston Globe*, September 21, 2012.

2. Ibid.

3. Amber J. Hammons et al., "Shared Family Meals Seem to Operate as a Protective Factor for Overweight, Unhealthy Eating, and Disordered Eating," *Pediatrics,* May 2011. "The Importance of Family Dinners VII," National Center on Addiction and Substance Abuse at Columbia University, June 2012.

INDEX